Dear Susan...
don't drink and decorate...
(a blueprint for the NHS?)

Len Bartholomew (LB)

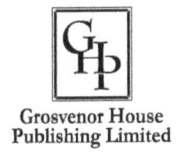

Grosvenor House
Publishing Limited

All rights reserved
Copyright © Len Bartholomew, 2023

The right of Len Bartholomew to be identified as the author of this
work has been asserted in accordance with Section 78
of the Copyright, Designs and Patents Act 1988

The book cover is copyright to Len Bartholomew

This book is published by
Grosvenor House Publishing Ltd
Link House
140 The Broadway, Tolworth, Surrey, KT6 7HT.
www.grosvenorhousepublishing.co.uk

This book is sold subject to the conditions that it shall not, by way of
trade or otherwise, be lent, resold, hired out or otherwise circulated
without the author's or publisher's prior consent in any form of
binding or cover other than that in which it is published and
without a similar condition including this condition being
imposed on the subsequent purchaser.

A CIP record for this book
is available from the British Library

ISBN 978-1-80381-501-5

Front and back cover – the beach and harbour wall - Greece

For Rosie (Rosemary (RG))

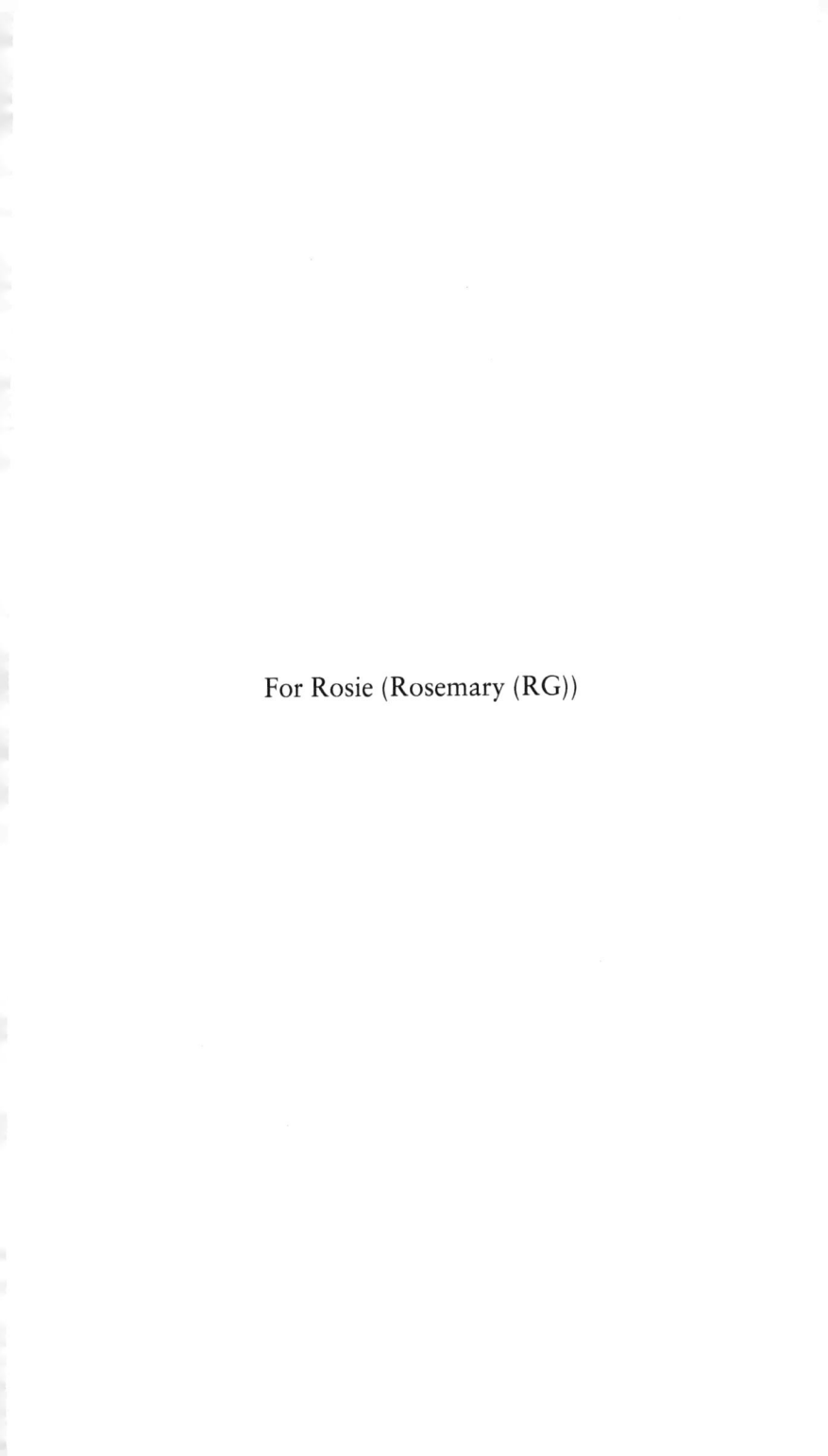

Foreword

For me and millions of people across the world, 2020 was the worst ever year. The first Covid 19 lockdown challenged us all to find ways to remain connected with our usual way of life. Our local NHS, even when it was not business-as-usual, chose to hold a public consultation with a closing date of 1st April 2020 about a proposal to build a large hospital in Sutton, Surrey. This was a red flag to a bull. LB could not believe plans developed pre-Covid could possibly be relevant to the needs of the NHS post-Covid, whenever that might be.

We got ourselves involved with writing to the Health and Social Care Committee and others, hoping that they too might have been thinking up new strategies for the NHS as it came to terms with the pandemic.

This post-retirement activity was further complicated later in 2020 by a need for LB to seek the help of a trauma team and inpatient care in a large NHS teaching hospital. From then on, there was no way to dampen his burning desire to comment about this experience to anybody who would listen and to make suggestions about what might be done to improve the patient experience. As this book shows, there is a need for the NHS to restore trust by improving its service for the health of the nation.

Fortunately, LB managed to retain his sense of humour with the help of 'Dear Susan,' the family WhatsApp group – 'don't drink and decorate.'friends, and some special people working for the NHS. Perhaps now that he has extracted this very large bee from his bonnet, while standing on one leg, he will allow us to get on with the rest of our lives and leave it all to someone else.

RG

February 2023

Preface

This book is my attempt to set out a blueprint for new NHS buildings, alongside my personal commentary about my experience as an inpatient in a large failing hospital, which highlighted some of the difficulties facing patients. This was during the NHS's struggle with the Covid-19 pandemic.

The buildings and facilities within which patients are treated and staff work, are so important to the wellbeing and successful outcomes for all concerned but are too often ignored. This book suggests a hospital building-led strategy to tackle the need for improvements for patients and staff. This approach was tried before, between 1970 and 1995. Then it was possible to show how new hospital buildings could promote change and innovation. Now is the time to try this again as the climate for change feels like that of the 1970s. A political will to sort out the NHS is essential.

The NHS and its staff are in desperate need for action – this really is the NHS's winter of discontent.

LB

February 2023

Contents

Introduction	1
Chapter 1 – The Long Road to Recovery	7
Chapter 2 – Dear Susan	17
Chapter 3 – Once Upon a Time Around 1970	29
Chapter 4 – Dear Mr Chairman - 1	37
Chapter 5 – Dear Chief Transformation Officer	49
Chapter 6 – "We will build 40 New Hospitals"	57
Chapter 7 – Dear Clare and Dear District Council	61
Chapter 8 – Dear Mr Chairman - 2	67
Chapter 9 – Dear Susan and Dear Mr Consultant	77
Chapter 10 – The Great Escape - May 2022	89
Chapter 11 – Dear Secretary of State	97
Chapter 12 – Enough Is Enough	101
Addendum – Fantasy Smaller Hospitals	107
Omission	115
A short letter to the RIBA Journal	117
Acknowledgements and Epitaph	119
A Last Word	123

Introduction

Ankle surgery – LB – Patient no. XXXXX – DOB 25/8/1941

This book is about an accidental fall requiring emergency hospital services during the first year of Covid at the end of November 2020. This is not about Covid – it is more about surviving the NHS after the ambulance is called to rush you off to hospital.

It is also about a few dedicated individuals working in a large failing hospital (due to be refurbished sometime). In passing, it shows how reluctant a local GP service had become to treat and counsel patients and was unable to provide crucial backup for overstretched hospital services. Also, that survival is a better bet with a family network in support.

In this case, the two over-performing services from November 2020 – the worst year of Covid – were the emergency ambulance and district nursing services. This came as a complete surprise. Following discharge from hospital, district nurses came to call for ten months, sometimes twice a week, to change dressings and to fight infections even when overloaded by patients not being allowed to see a GP. They always seemed to be able to put their patients' interest first. A very good local GP nursing service took over from the district nurses when they were allowed to resume face-to-face nursing in September 2021. This was without meaningful backup from GPs and only if a patient could get to the surgery.

The accidental fall from a stepladder occurred at home when final touches were being put to the decorating in a revamped bathroom. Ironically, the revamping was about ripping out a bath to provide a walk-in shower as it was becoming too difficult to step over the bath. The stepladder gave way and snapped shut on the right ankle as the decorator and the ladder fell to the floor. Two 'open' fractures resulted to each of the two bones between the knee and the ankle on impact. An open five-litre can of F&B Elephant's Breath paint (grey with a hint of pink) followed the fall to the floor, spilling over the upper part of the decorator's body.

The ambulance crew arrived within 30 minutes, removed clothing spreading the surplus paint evenly over the naked torso and stretchered the painted body to the ambulance. The two paramedics stabilised the trauma/ankle, administered morphine, and, most importantly, were reassuring about what was to follow. They tended the injury for half an hour parked up outside the house in readiness for a blue-light journey, in a past-its-sell-by-date ambulance to the nearest hospital – East Surrey Hospital, Redhill. Covid meant that it was a solo journey – leaving behind at home a shocked wife and the mess of a ruined brand new shower room.

At A&E, the team was waiting and ready on arrival. The handover by the ambulance crew was exemplary. One of the nurses asked if the dried Elephant's Breath coating was the patient's usual colour, a comment enjoyed by A&E staff gathered around the trolley. Orthopaedic surgery followed to further stabilise the ankle after it was decided that East Surrey Hospital was not equipped to fix this kind of severe trauma. Another blue-light ambulance was to make the journey to St George's Major Trauma Centre in Tooting. Again, the paramedics were timely, speedy, reassuring, and good-humoured. At St George's, in the early hours of the morning, the trauma centre team was waiting, as was the CT scanner. After another good handover by the ambulance crew it became clear to the orthopaedic senior registrar that the 'open' fractures and soft tissue damage was so severe that, without further surgery, it was looking like the lower leg below the knee might not be saved.

Early morning in a busy recovery ward saw the leg in a rigid metal rig looking realigned, which at first was a shock but seemed better than predicted. One needs to come-to in a recovery ward to see the NHS at its very best. It is only possible to guess about the contribution and skills of the anaesthetist, orthopaedic surgeons and theatre staff when viewing their work as you begin to recover and start to count your toes, legs, and blessings. The in and out movement of theatre trolleys in a busy recovery ward is in dreamlike slow motion in a strangely hushed and optimistic space as you are coaxed to take a drink and a sandwich to show you that you are still alive.

After recovery, life on a Covid-free orthopaedic ward is frenetic but bearable even without visitors. Isolation from Covid was helped by a WhatsApp group set up by the family called 'don't drink and decorate' (a tease!). This included the decorator/patient's wife, Rosie (Rosemary/RG), grown-up children and spouses/partners, and grandchildren. Providing regular finger-tapping answers to questions and concerns helped pass the time of day when the ward routine allowed. This continued into recovery at home.

As it happened the decorator/patient was a retired architect who had spent most of his working life specialising in the design of hospitals. He was able to do this without ever needing to sample life in hospital as an inpatient. Of course, hospital visits were necessary over many years to comfort family and friends or to oversee hospital building projects. He hoped that, by the time he retired, every hospital would be fit for purpose. He expected that at some time in the not-too-distant future, fewer large hospitals would be needed. These would be replaced by bright, shiny, optimistic, and therapeutic smaller hospitals with less staff doing so much more to mend/cure any condition/symptom and reduce the need for lengthy hospital admissions and invasive treatments – with many diagnoses and minor treatments being done online to bypass a failing GP service. Waiting lists would be a thing of the past – a responsive NHS.

Perhaps this was all wishful thinking when faced with a Covid pandemic but the 'shock-horror' experience of being referred to St George's confirmed the reality that the NHS was nowhere near providing the right kind of hospitals needed for the 2020s and the massive backlog caused by Covid could not be resolved without a drastic change of government policy.

December 2020 was a difficult month. St George's was a long way from home. Its major trauma centre covered a catchment area well beyond its location in South West London. Patients from Surrey and East and West Sussex were referred to St George's for complex orthopaedic procedures and Covid was out and about. During eight days as an inpatient, the external rigid metal rig was removed and replaced by internal metal parts during a third operation. The leg below the knee was encased in a plaster cast and the countdown for discharge began. The trauma team's physiotherapist and occupational therapists began deliberations about managing at home, as did a geriatrician. At home the wrecked shower room had been sorted, thanks to Matt the installer.

Discharge was agreed when the patient dressed himself and was seated in the bedside armchair in time for the ward round as if ready to go home. When it was shown that the patient could hop to the loo and back using a Zimmer, applauded by the other seven orthopaedic patients in the eight-bed bay, it was game on! What was not foreseeable was how the next two years would pan out.

The moral of this story is don't drink and decorate, don't use a Wickes stepladder when you are too old and too heavy, and don't wait until you are 79 before you need to experience trauma inpatient care for the very first time – during a Covid pandemic. Also, that the NHS needs all the help it can get to get through an almost unsolvable waiting list crisis and a few suggestions are floated here which describe a possible post-Covid blueprint for the NHS. In short, try to avoid

LB = DECORATOR/PATIENT

being admitted to hospital by looking after yourself and by making the right choices about everything likely to harm you. If you do ever need inpatient hospital care and the NHS is still in dire straits make sure you have a supportive WhatsApp group and your very own 'Dear Susan.'

Chapter 1
The Long Road to Recovery

Before the long road to recovery can be described it is necessary to dwell briefly the on time spent on the orthopaedic ward and the mark it leaves on some patients. H Ward was one of two 28-bed wards allocated to the Major Trauma Centre. It was comforting to realise that your trauma was fully understood by nursing staff familiar with the needs of orthopaedic patients. They were alert to all limited movements, difficulties in getting comfortable and the relief of pain. Day and night staff were readily available at the push of a button. Considering the multi-bed bay was shared by eight male patients with varying conditions and needs, the disruption was often lessoned by the business of nursing carried out mostly in a calm and relaxed manner. Dominic, nearest the nursing station, an 80- year-old jogger run over when a lorry mounted a curb behind him, found ward life difficult at times and clearly needed the specially arranged all-day visits from his son to help handle what Dominic felt was staff bullying, rather than assistance. Larry, next to the window and view, had fallen downstairs, seriously damaging his vertebrae and was not only in pain but was anxious about how he might ever manage at home when discharged, even though he had successfully arranged for the shattered stair balustrade to be repaired from his hospital bed. The styling of a made-to-measure straightjacket/spinal corset so concerned him that it was touch and go about his eventual discharge. A young Albanian man opposite had been in the hospital for months after he had received life-threatening injuries from a racial attack by a gang, which left him needing help from a whole range of hospital specialists. He was reluctant to speak, but would give you a thumbs-up when you asked him how he was doing. He was in a state of poverty, without prospect of work, homeless and unable to contemplate leaving hospital, which had become his safe haven. And so on... as patients came and went with rarely an empty bed.

Life on the ward was made difficult by the crowded, outdated nature of the facilities and the lack of space around beds. Given that visitors were not allowed, it was still difficult to find space to store aids and personal items without clutter making it impossible to clean, which was worrying in a pandemic. The ward layout was a long way from what was envisaged for future hospitals where many more single rooms with ensuites are now becoming the norm in new projects. For orthopaedic patients at St George's, the challenge was finding the loo, let alone using it, and if you managed to get there without a fall it was not unusual for its facilities to be occupied, with nowhere nearby to sit waiting for it to become free. Or it was out of use.

As you waited in your cubicle for the busy ward routine to run its course, it was easy to hope that discharge would come soon. However positive you are about your condition; it soon becomes clear that it is likely to worsen the longer you remain anchored to your bed or chair. Home begins to feel as if it might be a perfect aid to daily living and recovery because of its familiarity, close travel distances, brand new shower room, meal preferences, and your life is in your hands. The ward rounds do not provide an opportunity for you to discuss progress. These are mainly used for clinical staff and medical students to discuss amongst themselves what they think should be done with each patient. This exchange is difficult to follow as they could be talking about anyone. It can become fun if you can pitch a question at the professor, especially if you can think up one that cannot be answered – oh the joy of hearing a snigger from a medical student or, better still, a senior registrar.

Discharge came as a great relief. This, of course, was without a clue about the shape of things to come as an outpatient. When you are told that recovery could take a year, 18 months, or longer, you somehow think this must be the worst-case scenario. But it can get much worse.

During the eight days as an inpatient, the long haul to recovery began. This was going to be followed by many return visits to St George's. The first follow-up appointment was within two weeks in the orthopaedic clinic – ground floor, St James' Wing, if you can get there. This clinic was like a warzone. You took your turn to be called forward for an X-ray a long way down the hospital street or dispatched to a cramped, internal, airless, overheated, Covid-cleansed consulting room where you were left waiting until it suddenly became rammed full from a visitation by a masked trauma team. At least you were safe while set aside in the consultation room. All movement around the crowded clinic waiting space entailed squeezing past or stepping over resigned orthopaedic patients adorned with a variety of dressings, plaster casts, surgical boots, leg, arm, torso frames/irons, all of which are difficult to manoeuvre around without assistance and so easy to bump. And so on... Get the picture? Thankfully, this efficiently run clinic somehow ran to time. You were done and dusted and, on your way, wearing something new after calling by the plaster room to be fitted for a colour of your choice plaster cast or the latest air walker surgical boot, and then left all alone to retrieve your car before you realised you had not eaten your homemade sandwich.

By 6th July 2021, and after seven months of little progress and very little mobility, it was decided that 'salvage surgery' was needed on the lower leg and ankle. Internal metal plates were to be removed and instead an external fixator (invented by a Professor Ilizarov) was to be fitted. This entailed passing rods and wires through leg bones and bolting these to a substantial cylindrical metal frame clamping the four fractures together. Not a pleasant experience, requiring another ten days as an inpatient. After the operation, the recovery ward staff were calming and attentive although it was worrying to peer down the bed covers. The frame was not a pretty sight and made the leg look irreparable.

6th July 2021

WhatsApp group – don't drink and decorate

Hi all - some news. After an early 7am arrival (thanks to Beryl) Dad/Grandad went into surgery at 10am and came out at 4:30. A very long haul. He is still in the recovery ward but will be transferred later to V Ward –what an ordeal for him! Love to all, Rosie.

Unlike the first inpatient experience, this second inpatient stay was going to prove to be more of a challenge. Transfer from the recovery ward was to V Ward a 'green' (Covid-free) former ENT ward. Here, nurses were unfamiliar with mobility issues experienced by orthopaedic patients. They were less alert and less patient about patients needing to pee or use a commode, they would store away crutches and Zimmer's, which needed to be on-hand, and they would be irritated by patients who dared push the nurse call buzzer. The trauma team ward round did not visit you because their patient was not on the orthopaedic ward where they expected him to be.

6th July 2021

WhatsApp group: from decorator/patient

Tucked up! in 8-bed dorm on V Ward with 7 other football-watchers and 7 other potential snorers in time to watch the penalty shootout. Love to all.

This ward provided a revolving door admission of patients with wide-ranging needs. The ward layout was like the orthopaedic ward but somehow its layout presented staff with more problems. Some patients were returnees who, over many visits, seemed to have become so familiar with the hospital routine that they chose to help themselves. An empty bed opposite was taken by an 18-year-old man who walked into the eight-bed bay, introduced himself, and staked his claim by dumping his belongings on a vacant bed. He timed his admission until after the meal trolley had come and gone. He then popped down to M&S in the main entrance to buy a snack bag. He had had sickle cell issues for most of his young life but had educated himself at home and was anticipating gaining a place at Oxford. He was a breath of fresh air who, within six hours, was trollied off never to return to our ward, having been given a different berth elsewhere in the hospital – lucky him.

His bed was filled by John, another returnee, readmitted to have his two hip replacements serviced as he had almost become immobile. A cheeky chappie character, working in ventilation, who knew his way around the ward and seemed to know every member of staff. John was the most well-equipped patient ever, with everything to hand including iPad, Netflix, bed socks, an electric toothbrush, and emergency snacks. He made sure the ward lights were left on so all eight patients were awake for the Euros final – right up to the penalty shootout – and was probably responsible for the extra tea and biscuits served just before lights out. John was also responsible for diverting patients from thinking about their ailments during the match and their depression after Italy won. Many other patients came and went...

Life on the ward at the time of the Euros could not disguise the fact that the ward was out of date, drab, crowded, uncomfortable, too noisy and the multi-bed bay had too many beds. It badly needed refurbishment. The NHS and its patients deserve better – it is difficult to gauge just how much these facilities affect patient outcomes and staff morale – who has time to care?

7th July 2021

WhatsApp group: from decorator/patient

Thanks for today's text messages, lovely Jane, Jo and Lauren, and all other lovelies for so many cheering and uplifting messages. Last night amongst the 8 snorers was made interesting wondering who might get through the night and how many times the air ambulance would land on the roof above my top-floor dorm – which fortunately happened only once. The building just about held together! Now waiting for the ward round to find out more. Love to all.

7th July 2021

WhatsApp group: from decorator/patient

Still waiting for the ward round, lovely Lauren, Anna and Jane. I'm not on the ortho ward but in the ENT ward so could be last or lost.

7th July 2021

WhatsApp Group: from decorator/patient

Hi all lovelies – an orthopaedic senior registrar turned up at 5pm along with my supper of meatballs and carrots followed by orange jelly (yuk!). He promptly checked my ears, nose and throat and said the op went well although tricky and long. They have fitted an external, temporary, metal cylinder to hold them bones, them bones... together until the next outpatient clinic yet to be fixed. Tomorrow they are helping me to transfer weight to the ankle. Now for the penalty shootout! Hugs to all.

Getting discharged was proving difficult. It was conditional on the need for an intravenous course of antibiotics tailored to knock out the bacteria found at the infected site. This was to be managed at home through daily visits from a member of the home care team who needed to be programmed to avoid coming at the same time as the district nurses. The decorator/patient had to have a 'PICC line' inserted by the X-ray department so a daily bag of antibiotics could be connected at each home visit.

Discharge was achieved on 16th July 2021. The next two months living with Prof Ilizarov's fixator was uncomfortable. The district nurses continued to clean and dress the 'pins' penetrating the leg at 14 puncture points to keep infections at bay. This could take up to an hour each visit but, again, the district nurses came up trumps. On the occasions when they became concerned about the condition of the leg, they contacted the GP and when not satisfied with the response would email St George's for advice. If they thought additional home visits were necessary, they somehow juggled their schedules. The district nurses stood down on 11th September so the GP nurses could take the baton and run with the nursing care. There was one significant moment before the handover when, on 23rd August, one of the pins passing through the ankle snapped, which was promptly reported to the trauma team. It was removed at the 2nd September clinic and replaced under full anaesthetic at day surgery on 14th September. Shortly after, another pin snapped. At the Orthoplastic clinic on 21st October 2021, it was decided to abort the 'fixator' as it seemed the leg was rejecting the intrusion and infection was increasingly difficult to control. It was removed under full anaesthetic on 9th November at day surgery.

And on and on! The long road to recovery was to take more than two years, which seemed forever. This was to bleed hospital resources during the pandemic and beyond. So far, it has taken six operations, three inpatient admissions, 13 visits to the X-ray department and outpatient attendances. One year after the fall, at the 18th November 2021 Orthoplastic clinic, the consultants gave the decorator/patient a 50:50 chance of saving or losing his leg below the right knee – a loud reaction could not budge these odds. On the 16th December 2021, the odds improved in favour of saving the leg to 65:35, 80:20 on 20th January 2022, and 90:10 on the 17th March 2022. On the 5th May 2022, they were 95:5 and these odds remain to this day – eureka with a limp!

Chapter 2
Dear Susan

So where does 'Dear Susan' fit in? Dear Susan is the secretary to three consultant orthopaedic surgeons at St George's Hospital. Contact came about after the family's dear Jo, also a consultant's secretary but in a private hospital, could see that in order to get to the heart of the matter of survival as an in or outpatient in any large hospital, there was no point in dealing with anyone but the consultant's secretary. As it turned out, the 'Patient Portal' is the worst possible way for a patient to communicate with the NHS. It is pointless trying to phone, text, or email clinical, admin staff, or patient group volunteers because everyone is too busy to respond. Hospital secretaries command the airways, have the patients' notes to hand, and can communicate with staff in all departments. More importantly, they manage their consultants. Clinical/medical staff have their hands full dealing with patients in the flesh in a face-to-face or any other body part moment. That same face, after that moment, becomes faceless as soon as another patient is wheeled in to the consulting/treatment space.

The patient's body part, name, hospital number, date of birth is the defining confirmation of who a patient

LB = DECORATOR/PATIENT

is – at first printed on unremovable wrist bands and thereafter on all correspondence. Visual identification is further complicated when everyone is wearing a mask. The masked decorator/patient did not see his orthopaedic or plastics consultants and their senior registrars without masks for 18 months after discharge. He could have walked past them without being recognised or recognising them. In this case, it is not clear whether an exaggerated hop or limp and a Zimmer helped recognition.

A few emails were exchanged with the senior orthopaedic registrar, Zoe, in March 2021. Zoe was on-hand in the early hours of the morning of 26th November 2020 when the decorator/patient was transferred to St George's A&E department still coated in Elephant's Breath paint. Zoe has a wonderful bedside manner, even with bad news, and was usually on-hand for ward rounds and at clinic appointments until she was moved from 'ankles' to 'elbows' after six months. Zoe was one the of few people in the hospital able to see emails as a useful way to communicate with patients. Also, Zoe copied in 'Dear Susan' so 'Dear Susan' was unearthed – she is the secretary to the ankle specialist consultant allocated to the decorator/patient – but more about 'Dear Susan' later. Her contribution is recorded for posterity in this book.

From discharge on 3rd December 2020 until 4th March 2021 there was no need to email Dear Zoe, Dear Susan, or anyone else. Real time contact as an outpatient was frequent in December – with two before Christmas and a third visit to the clinic on December 29th, but progress seemed slow in the new year after another Orthoplastic clinic on 7th January 2021. GP services were non-existent even though St George's needed local services to cover patients who were too far away from the hospital's local South West London catchment area. As mentioned earlier, the district nurses continued throughout Covid to plug the breach against the odds with an increase in referrals when patients were no longer able to see a GP. At the 7th January clinic, it was suggested that weight should not be transferred to the damaged ankle until the next appointment on 4th March, even when wearing an air walker surgical boot. The idea being, in lay terms, that the boot would hold the foot onto the leg while the fractures grew together and the damaged complex ankle soft tissues could find a way to regenerate and heal. The boot was removable for care and attention of the incisions and open wound. The advice was to wear it continuously, even in bed, elevated on pillows. It was to be worn in bed should it be necessary to get up during the night to prevent further damage from knocking the ankle loose in the dark on the way to the loo. The district nurses were to continue home visits to change dressings and to keep an eye on things during a long waiting game for the ankle to start to recover. The first Covid jab came on stream on 23rd January 2021 to relieve the feeling of being a sitting duck with no place to run.

As the realities began to sink in, a message was posted on 23rd December 2020 to the WhatsApp group 'don't drink and decorate' from the decorator/patient.

> We have just got home from another long day at the Orthoplastic (orthopaedic and plastics combined) clinic. Between them it could be positive to have two competing powers of healing. They seem to agree that I might have been pulled back from the brink! I put it down to your love and support, prayers, Rosie's tender loving care and Jane's gun powder tablets (ssshhhh!) taken as told. We left St George's with a course of penicillin and a new boot, which looks like a boot Greek sponge divers wear to descend to the depths off Kalymnos. We have to return to St George's on 29th December to plan next steps. So yippee, we are at home at Christmas like the rest of you, unless we decide to go sponge fishing!

Amongst the many supportive replies was one from Will:

> Brilliant news, Grandad, so pleased to hear that. Now put your feet up both and have a great Christmas and no sponge diving!

And another from niece Beryl:

> That's great news, Uncle. Looks like rattling the gates of heaven worked!

The 4th March X-ray was more encouraging and the Orthoplastic team suggested it was time to gradually transfer weight to the damaged leg and to get off the bed and walk until the next appointment on 16th April.

Things took a slight upturn until 23rd March. It was then that a need to have someone to email at St George's became clearer.

24th March 2021

Email to Mr Consultant from decorator/patient

Dear Mr Consultant

We last spoke when I attended your outpatient clinic on 4th March. You advised me to begin to transfer weight to my ankle cautiously, to continue with visits by the district nurse to manage the 'open wound' and to attend your clinic again on 6th May.

For three weeks now, I have been walking around my home unaided but wearing the surgical boot or without the boot with a Zimmer, alternating as need be – not an ambitious programme.

The district nurse called yesterday – 23rd March – and she expressed concern about swelling around the ankle opposite the healing open wound and a build-up of water around the wounds and your incisions. There is no leakage at present but the swelling is causing numbness and tenderness. Do I need to ask my GP to prescribe water tablets to reduce swelling and face the subsequent need for blood tests to monitor their effect or is this swelling a usual outcome of loading the ankle as part of the recovery process? Photos will be forwarded separately by email.

So far I have been unable to connect with any physiotherapy guidance although I do have a telephone call booked to speak to my GP practice physiotherapist on 12th April.

Many thanks

LB = DECORATOR/PATIENT

25th March 2021

Email to Dear Susan, cc Zoe, from decorator/patient

Dear Susan

Can you please ensure that Mr Consultant sees the above email and the photographs emailed to him separately? I regard this as urgent business.

Thank you

25th March 2021

Email from Zoe to decorator/patient

Dear LB

I can't see any photos, please could you send them to me?

Many thanks

30th March 2021

Email to Zoe from decorator/patient

Sorry to email you again before you have had a chance to talk with Mr Consultant following recent exchanges. I was half-expecting that on reviewing my next clinic date scheduled for the 6th May you might have considered bringing this forward. However, yesterday I received a letter dated 25th March from outpatient appointments cancelling 6th May and offering me another on 3rd June. Does this make any sense to you?

Kind regards

31st March 2021

Email from Zoe to decorator/patient

Dear LB

Mr Consultant agrees we need to see you sooner than June so we will ask our secretary to bring forward that appointment. Did you get anywhere with the physio?

Best wishes

31st March 2021

Email to Zoe from decorator/patient

Dear Zoe

Many thanks for your email. Re. physiotherapy, as far as I know. my situation remains unchanged. It seems that my gateway into NHS physiotherapy services is still via a telephone conversation with my GP practice physiotherapist scheduled for 9am on 12th April.

Kind regards

At the Orthoplastic clinic on 29th April 2021 it was confirmed that the ankle was infected between the bone and splint and that 'salvage' surgery might be necessary. At the 3rd June 2021 clinic, after a three-week course of antibiotics and a scan it was confirmed that more surgery was needed if it could be scheduled.

LB = DECORATOR/PATIENT

25th June 2021

Email to Dear Susan from decorator/patient

Dear Susan

Three weeks ago, Mr Consultant explained that I needed urgent 'salvage' surgery to adjust previous surgery to my right ankle carried out by the trauma team at the end of November 2020. I understood that urgent meant in 4-6 weeks' time and that doing nothing to my ankle was not an option.

I have been in touch with admissions... in order to plan tests for Covid 19 prior to being admitted. I was told I am on a waiting list... My prospects for urgent corrective surgery seem to be diminishing.

It is now seven months since my initial surgery. I am still non-ambulant requiring a surgical boot for support to cover very short distances and my ankle is painful when I transfer load with or without the boot.

I appreciate that St George's, like all hospitals, has a long waiting list... but I would appreciate knowing from Mr Consultant how long is reasonable to wait for the surgery he has in mind... for me, a delay resulting in a deterioration in the condition of my ankle and lower leg would be the worst outcome.

Kind regards

An admission date of 6th July 2021 was fixed for 'salvage' surgery requiring up to ten days as an inpatient.

7th July 2021

Email to Dear Susan from decorator/patient

Dear Susan

After yesterday's surgery I was admitted to V... ENT Ward. Is it likely that I have missed out on the orthopaedic team's ward round today? It is now 4pm and I was hoping to have advice and feedback about how I manage my condition and start to move about!

Many thanks

An orthopaedic registrar who had assisted with the operation arrived at the bedside at 5pm.

13th July 2021

Email to Dear Susan from decorator/patient

Dear Susan

I'm afraid it's me again. At Monday's ward round I was expecting to be told that I could be discharged having spent six nights in hospital.

We discussed a delay to the microbiologist results of samples taken from the wound site on the day of my operation. Lead Consultant asked his team to chase up these results. I explained that I was ready to be discharged because I felt I could better manage to home-care my condition and the external structure now clamping my fractured bones... I can no longer see a need for me to remain on a ward where increasingly the needs of more recent admissions outweigh my own.

Lead Consultant suggested that I should talk this over with Mr Consultant today. Today's ward round without him confirmed that he is unlikely to be available soon as Tuesday is his theatre list day. Therefore, I would be grateful if you could please let him know how I feel about discharge. As I see it, I am remaining in hospital only for the purpose of taking a general antibiotic until the microbiologist can design one specifically for my treatment. It is not obvious to me why either of these two antibiotics should not be prescribed for home use. Today's ward round indicated that a 'PICC line' needs to be inserted before I leave hospital to intravenously feed antibiotics at home. Could this be put in hand soon?

Thanks for your help

13th July 2021

Email from Dear Susan to decorator/patient

I have let Mr Consultant know for you and he will discuss later when he sees you.

Susan

Sure enough, and to my surprise, Mr Consultant and his senior registrar appeared at my bedside within the hour in surgical gowns following a lull in their theatre list. I was to remain on this ward for another four days.

The above emails give a flavour of the email trail over the next 18 months. They are included here and in later chapters to show how these were used to seek help and to make a point about how things were not working. Also, to make suggestions about how things might be improved when the NHS clearly was in crisis – a kind of payback for the treatment being provided. It seemed that a sitting duck might see things differently about what could be done from a traumatised patient perspective.

The decorator/patient/retired architect was well placed to see how things might need to change. Whether this simple belief was more to do with the trauma, the ageing process, or just because of a need for something to do to while away the time is anyone's guess.

Chapter 3

Once Upon a Time Around 1970

Way back in the distant past, around the early 1970s, serious thought was being given about how the Victorians could build so many hospitals in such a short time and why, since 1948, when the NHS came about, it seemed to take forever.

The Minister of State for Health at the Department of Health was seeking action that might drastically reduce the time it was taking to plan and build new hospitals and prevent the massive time and construction cost overruns that were a common occurrence. Also, he wanted to know more about a programme of standardised hospitals for a rapidly changing and uniform NHS to replace the Victorian and pre-war legacies.

At that time there was little thought given to the consequences of achieving rapid build hospitals and about how they might be managed and staffed. It was enough to show that it could be done. No one thought it would be possible to build hospitals faster than it would be to train or recruit staff or whether it would ever be possible to afford to replace all those hospitals that were no longer fit for purpose in a shorter time frame.

LB = DECORATOR/PATIENT

So, a discussion between the health minister, the chief works officer and the chief architect kick-started the largest ever, nationally controlled, hospital-building programme. Probably the largest building project of any kind anywhere apart from the Great Wall of China.

To tackle the task, a third of a central London skyscraper was used to house a team of over 150 doctors, nurses, administrators, researchers, engineers, quantity surveyors and architects. They were to focus their minds on delivering the nucleus hospital briefing and design system. They were assisted by teams in 14 regional health authorities across the country who would be responsible for commissioning nucleus hospitals in each region. Many private practice architects and engineers would design and arrange tenders for hospitals tailored to meet local service planning priorities. It was a huge undertaking using a simple planning concept. Standard hospital departments were planned in a cruciform template – hospital Lego blocks – that could be assembled to form the nucleus/part of a whole hospital. For example, four operating theatres, support rooms, and a recovery ward were planned to fit into one cruciform template. This same template could house two 28-bed wards, and so on.

For new hospitals, a first phase 'nucleus' might use 12-16 cruciform templates with six to eight on each of two floors, providing up to 300 beds. A hospital providing 300 beds, the size of a district general hospital serving a local catchment area of 250,000 people, could be expanded to provide up to 600 beds. The cruciform template, in rows either side of a hospital street, allowed for natural lighting and ventilation[1] and was intended to be used for two- and at most three-story solutions. The templates could also be used as an addition to an existing hospital.

The architectural profession loved or hated nucleus. Some practices resented only being commissioned to construct and elevate hospitals using standard data. Others were pleased to be informed about specialised aspects of hospital planning and design and contributed hugely to the provision of hospitals fit for rapidly changing treatment procedures. Prior to nucleus, the notion that each hospital should be unique and reflect a new opportunity to reinvent what a hospital should be had resulted in some being costly and unworkable – some have been demolished perhaps prematurely. Some nucleus hospitals were disappointing but others were inspirational. They all consistently worked for the staff using them.

In 1991, a published review indicated that 28 new nucleus hospitals had been commissioned. This type of hospital continued to be built for another ten years after the chief architect retired in 1993.

Ironically, or befittingly, the chief works officer and chief architect, who joined forces with the health minister to give birth to nucleus, both lived in Reigate and were to see out their last days in East Surrey

---

[1] In 1990, a low-energy nucleus hospital was show to use 50% less energy than older hospitals, helped by natural lighting and ventilation, and its cruciform templates.

LB = DECORATOR/PATIENT

Hospital, Redhill – one of the first nucleus hospitals to be commissioned. It was a close call for the decorator/patient/retired architect when he was transferred from the same local hospital to St George's Major Trauma Centre.

Eventually over 150 were built of all sizes using the cruciform template, which, over time, was revised internally to incorporate changing standards. Of course, nucleus had its downside. Some of the nucleus hospitals built were too large, in the wrong place, and are now in need of upgrading. However, many of them are still much better than most of the one-offs built before or at the same time.

The Covid pandemic, the resulting chaos, and the need to clear a massive backlog of patient operations has left the NHS wanting a new generation of rapidly built hospital buildings. Unfortunately, there does not seem to be anybody around with a political will to make this happen.

Nucleus hospitals will serve the NHS for a few more years yet but they were not designed to deal with the backlog caused by Covid. Something different is needed to fix the NHS but it is not by building one or two mega-hospitals or by attempting to transform large existing hospitals like St George's.

In providing rapidly built nucleus hospitals in the 1970s, '80s and '90s, it was argued that these should replace or improve Victorian and pre- and post-Second World War hospitals when it might have been more appropriate to set out a new service plan for the nation's health care needs. Some nucleus hospitals were built alongside existing hospitals where it was soon clear that they should have been located elsewhere. However, from the conveyor belt of new nucleus hospitals, a few were set aside to be built to stand alone on newly acquired sites. When this happened, it was possible to reflect on a new beginning for the NHS.

New, easy, fast, smart, smaller hospitals could provide the next generation of hospitals. All that is needed is for someone in the NHS to want to build one to shine the light in the current darkness. How this might work is dealt with later in subsequent chapters. It stems from a notion that would leave existing NHS hospitals as they are for the time being and to only build new hospitals specialising in either trauma emergency care – for which there seems to be an ever-present need – or elective care to efficiently deal with the waiting list backlog, handling procedures that can be done in a day. These would be self-sufficient stand-alone hospitals built quickly to cause an impact. Existing hospitals would continue to be used for all other specialties – upgraded where obvious.

In 1975 the health minister was trying to get a grip on building new hospitals in 'the difficult economic circumstances of the next few years[2]'. He was wanting to encourage the development and use of nucleus hospitals with a standardised but flexible basic design

---

[2] Extracts from a 1975 keynote speech made by the Minister of Health.

of around 300 beds. 'Large district general hospitals built in one phase were no longer feasible.' More fundamentally, he thought that 'by building for the essential, not the desirable, number of beds, one can spread the limited capital resources and start more new hospital development'. Also, 'in the absence of growth and the presence of high Inflation, capital restriction will be greater than anyone would wish over the next few years.'

This look back at once upon a time around 1970 strangely fits the context of today following the Covid pandemic. It could also be argued today that we should not be building hospitals as large as 300 beds. Large hospitals are from the past and things need to move on – the decorator/patient/retired architect found his time at St George's a painful flashback.

DEAR SUSAN... DON'T DRINK AND DECORATE...

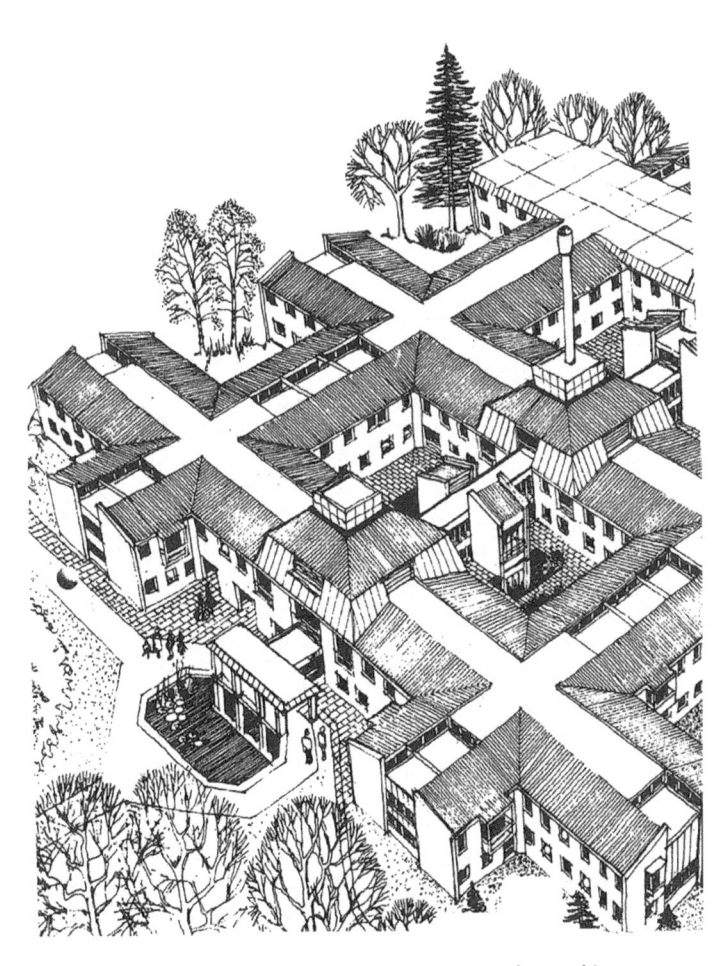

Standard hospital departments were planned in
a cruciform template – hospital Lego blocks.

Chapter 4
Dear Mr Chairman - 1

Sometime before St George's Major Trauma Centre became a preoccupation, and during the first Covid lockdown in 2020, there was a public consultation about a proposal to build a large new hospital in Sutton, Surrey. The lockdown and the NHS response to the pandemic provided the opportunity to think about what kind of hospitals might be needed for the 2020s after Covid.

Planned over many years before Covid, this proposal for a large new hospital, if accepted, was likely to be the first hospital to be built after Covid – even though a fairer distribution of scarce resources should now be a real concern for the NHS. Following the public consultation, a brochure was produced by two local residents (LB and RG) to illustrate a different approach. This was sent to the chief executive, Epsom & St Heller University Hospitals NHS Trust, the local MP, and Opinion Research Services.[3] It was also forwarded to the chair of the Health and Social Care Select

---

[3] It seems reasonable to record that some of these people were too busy to acknowledge or reply to a hard copy brochure posted to them by recorded delivery or to subsequent emails – except Opinion Research Services for Surrey Downs, Sutton and Merton local NHS and the chairman of the Health and Social Care Parliamentary Select

Committee. Surely this committee would have a view about what now might be needed?

29th May 2020

Email to Opinion Research Services from local residents LB and RG

Dear Team

Please find the attached brochure, which we have prepared to supplement our comments made in emails and your questionnaire for the Public Consultation for Surrey Downs, Sutton and Merton Local NHS.

Please note its distribution.

Yours sincerely

LB and RG

3rd June 2020

Email to LB and RG from Opinion Research Services

Dear LB and RG

A brief note of thanks for sending us a copy of your brochure. Your suggestions with regard to an alternative approach of building four smaller specialist emergency care hospitals[4] were noted during analysis of the questionnaire feedback and written submissions and are included, in summary form (with verbatim quotes), in our report and the appendix

---

Committee. Our local MP had no view on the matter, even when prompted on numerous occasions – oh dear!

[4] This ignores the point made in the brochure that it would be preferable to build one smaller hospital to start with and to only build more when the case is proven.

specifically highlighting alternative suggestions... I have forwarded the document to the IHT Programme team so they are aware of the source material and can disseminate it appropriately.

Kind regards

Charlie

8th June 2020

Email to Dear Charlie from LB and RG

Dear Charlie

Thank you for acknowledging receipt of our brochure and for tipping us off about the publication of your report with its appendix on alternative suggestions. This is a well-presented report which clearly shows how the consultation exercise backs the provision of a large SEC Hospital on the Sutton site.

The local bias against this from the community served by St Heller and, to a lesser degree, Epsom is perfectly understandable and we are interested to note that another site might be available at West Park...

Your report will help to encourage a 'pause for thought' given the circumstances we all face with Covid-19.

Kind regards

LB and RG

LB = DECORATOR/PATIENT

29th May 2020

Letter to chair of Health and Social Care Committee, House of Commons from LB and RG

Dear Chairman

New Smaller 2020 Hospitals

Just before Covid-19 locked down the country and put the NHS on red alert, a local NHS in Surrey Downs, Sutton and Merton was allocated £500 million to invest in hospital buildings. Its public consultation closed on 1st April 2020. This local NHS is now about to build a new 300-bed hospital at Sutton.

However, the Coronavirus outbreak has shown a need to think outside the box and to be more innovative in the provision of hospital facilities across the NHS.

The attached brochure attempts to paint a picture of what a new, smaller, 2020 hospital might be like as a more affordable alternative to large-scale provision.

We put this together during the lockdown and we hope this might make a difference in a wider context to improve the NHS.

Yours sincerely

LB and RG

1st July 2020

Email to chair of HSCC from LB and RG

Dear HSCC

Correspondence re. 2020 hospitals

We wrote to your chairman on 29th May enclosing a brochure re. easy, fast, smart, smaller 2020 hospitals to improve the NHS after Covid-19...

Is it unreasonable for us to expect a response within five weeks from the addressees? Even if they do not have the time or inclination to address its contents, might they at least acknowledge receipt?

LB and RG

4th July 2020

Email from chair of HSCC to LB and RG

Dear Mr LB and Ms RG

Thank you for your letter of 29 May regarding your proposal for the building of four smaller specialist emergency care hospitals (SECH) in your local area. In response to the recent consultation by Surrey Downs Sutton and Merton CCGs on a new local hospital. Thanks also for your follow-up email of 1 July.

I note that a decision is due to be made this week, and am very sorry for the delay in responding to that initial letter. As I am sure you will understand, my office has needed to make adjustments to the way it usually works during the COVID-19 period, which can unfortunately result in delays when responding to letters in hard copy.

Thank you for the work and thought that has gone into your proposals. I particularly appreciate you sharing learning from your experience as former employees of the Department of Health. The role of the Health and Social Care Committee is to scrutinise the administration, expenditure, and policy of the Department of Health and its associated public bodies. As such, it would be inappropriate for me to intervene in a particular case in my role as chair of the Committee.

However, as you may know, the Committee has been holding an inquiry on the delivery of core NHS and care services during the pandemic and beyond. The inquiry is looking at the question of whether and how the delivery of core services will have to change in the aftermath of COVID-19, and I believe that your ideas around the future of care in hospitals may have broader relevance to this topic. As such, I will bear your suggestions in mind as we consider the wider evidence we have received.

Once again, thank you for getting in touch.

Best wishes,

Chair, Health and Social Care Committee

House of Commons I London I SW1A OAA

May 18th 2021

Email to chair of HSCC from LB and RG

Dear Chairman

It is nearly a year since we forwarded you a hard copy of our brochure, New Smaller 2020 Hospitals, on 29th May 2020.

On receiving your reply of 4th July, we thought we should stand back and let your committee and others better placed than us decide what kind of hospitals would be required in the future. We felt we had done all we could do in responding *to our local public consultation, especially as our own MP and our local NHS had shown no interest in acknowledging or contributing to our brochure. We still strongly believe that our local NHS, on concluding its public consultation in March 2020 and being allocated central government funding soon after, should have reviewed its preferred option to build a large 300-bed hospital at Sutton.*

So, what has happened since to make us want to email you again? We unexpectedly needed the help of the NHS. In November 2020 one of us became a 'blue light' trauma patient admitted in the first instance to our local East Surrey Hospital and subsequently transferred to St George's Major Trauma Centre for specialist surgery. While receiving an exceptional level of inpatient care from the trauma team at St George's, we experienced first-hand the mismatch between the quality of care skilled staff are expected and able to achieve with the latest equipment but in the worst kind of hospital facilities. The trauma team urgently needs an opportunity to carry out its complex surgical procedures, and the processes of long-term recovery through inpatient and outpatient care, in facilities designed for this purpose. Currently the St George's trauma team is flying by the seat of its pants!

You will know that in 2017, St George's was under special measures and was charged to take on board performance recovery for quality and finance. Efforts have been underway since then to save, recover, maintain, and grow the hospital. St George's, like our local NHS and many other hospitals across the country, has had a large team planning for change over the last three years to radically update its failing hospital. It has a five-year plan to implement although the pandemic has rendered such long-term plans unaffordable and unfit for purpose. The possibility of a new standalone smaller 2020s Major Trauma Centre at St George's is a nonstarter because the five-year plan is set in concrete.

LB = DECORATOR/PATIENT

Surely, now gone are the days of long-term planning cycles and public consultations, leading to gradual and begrudging ways to improve existing hospitals like St George's, or the provision of large new monolithic, inflexible health care buildings like the one about to be built in Sutton. These are guaranteed to become a burden for decades, like St George's is now. The only justification for continuing this long, drawn-out planning process is to delay and hinder the provision of replacement hospitals in order to ration scarce central capital funding. Covid-19 demands that we urgently change this mind set.

We believe we have reached a time when, realistically, the provision of new hospitals must be limited by capping allocations for all local NHS capital projects. This should be seen as a positive policy. A way to achieve this would be to inform local NHSs that they can bid for a new smaller starter hospital of up to 10,000 sq. metres if they can demonstrate that this would foster a radical new approach to its service provision, including if possible, at an alternative location to their existing hospital. Existing. hospitals were probably built in the right place for the 1900s but are most likely to be in the wrong place for the 2020s. A strategy providing a network of smaller hospitals would make land acquisition easier.

A rapid construction programme should also be a condition of funding. We are imagining the production of brand new smaller, starter hospitals to kick-start a revitalised hospital construction Initiative. Local NHSs who successfully complete one smaller starter hospital could be allocated funds for a second if it can demonstrate a progressive approach and an enhanced performance.

Stockpiles of data and guidance exists to inform how smaller starter hospitals might be planned, designed, and commissioned in the 2020s. The solutions used in our brochure were based on this wealth of information. What is needed now is someone to sanction one smaller starter hospital prototype, or even better, a network of five. An enthusiastic NHS team, helped by one of our top ten architects not tainted by hospital design experience and selected from a limited competition, could plan, design and arrange manufacture. When the hospital is fully operational, they could monitor and compare its performance and advise local NHSs bidding for their own smaller starter hospital.

The pandemic has shown that we can learn to move quickly to provide the NHS with the equipment and temporary facilities staff demanded for their own hospitals when facing a relentless call for action. They did not want to use those oversized, wasteful, and nightmarish Nightingale hospitals! It has also shown that new and better facilities are urgently required to tackle the worrying waiting lists that are a consequence of the pandemic.

To summarize, a new smaller, starter hospital should be in the right location probably away from, but used in conjunction with, an existing hospital, be assembled quickly, be affordable within a fixed capital cost (up to l0,000 sq. metres in size) and have more relevance to the way clinical teams will have to work in the future. It should also be uncomplicated, understandable, therapeutic, flexible, and intensively used. When, over time, it reaches its sell-by date and becomes inflexible and obstructive, it should be able to be decommissioned, deconstructed, and replaced without fuss.

Now is the time to showcase how adaptable smaller starter hospitals can be provided quickly to replace our many failing hospitals. This would lift morale, renew confidence, and promote even better services throughout the NHS. A primary aim should be to demonstrate that the NHS will require less beds, not more, through improved performances in the right kind of facilities in the aftermath of this life-changing pandemic.

Is there any way in which your committee can encourage the development of smaller hospital units before more capital monies are allocated to the provision of mega hospitals, repeating the mistakes of the past?

Kind regards

LB and RG

August 19th 2021

Email from Chair HSCC to LB and RG

Dear Mr LB and Ms RG

Thank you for your email of 18 May regarding the development of smaller hospital units. I am sorry for the delay in replying at what has been an exceptionally busy time for the committee.

You mention the experience that one of you had last November at St George's as a trauma patient. I do hope that your recovery is going well. Your email also makes a number of interesting points about the scale of facilities the NHS will need going forwards. Unfortunately, the committee's forward programme is currently full. However, you may be Interested to know that we have recently begun an inquiry into clearing the backlog caused by the pandemic. You can find out more about the inquiry here. Submissions that address any or all of the call for evidence are welcome, and can be made here by 3 September.

Once again, thank you for getting in touch.

Best wishes

Chair, Health and Social Care Committee

House of Commons, London

This last email hinted at an opportunity to submit written evidence to the Health and Social Care Committee for its latest enquiry. This would take some effort from LB and RG but there was still time and they had no particular place to go. Also, at that time, it seemed that nobody else was doing too much about anything, which is probably still the case.

Chapter 5
Dear Chief Transformation Officer

As the decorator/patient/retired hospital architect had so much time on his hands and was not going anywhere, lying about with his leg elevated, it is not surprising that he began to want to dare tell those working at St George's what he thought of the place and how to reorganise and redevelop their hospital – but would anyone listen?

An opportunity arose one Orthoplastic clinic appointment day on 7th January 2021. The decorator/patient was seated in an immovable hospital wheelchair in the draughty main foyer near M&S, waiting for the car to be parked up somewhere, wondering if he would ever get to the Orthoplastic clinic on time. A hospital notice board came into focus on the opposite wall. It was the 'who's who', including portrait photographs of the whole hospital management team. This was more closely examined when a flustered Rosie arrived as it was easier for her to steer straight at the notice board than it was to push and turn the wheelchair to join the masked throng dutifully keeping to the two lanes set out on the floor to maintain the safe distances demanded by Covid. Much to our surprise, this included a photograph of our local district counsellor. He was also the 'chief transformation officer'! His task was to transform St George's Hospital from a failing hospital into a hospital fit for today. Not an easy task!

At the Orthoplastic clinic, the plaster cast had been exchanged for a surgical boot/air walker and we were advised to put nil weight on the booted ankle for the next two months. We left the clinic depressed about this outcome. On our way back to the car park we stopped the wheelchair to look again at the management portraits and decided there and then to email the chief transformation officer benignly smiling down at us:

19th January 2021

Email to Dear Chief Transformation Officer from LB and RG

Dear James

During the first lockdown, we produced a brochure which set out to rethink the size, location, and design of health care buildings from 2020 onwards, following a public consultation held by our local NHS. We sent this to our local MP but have yet to receive a reply or acknowledgement. We did get a very helpful reply from the HSCC in July 2020.

Recently, we needed to use the services of St George's University Hospitals Major Trauma Centre for emergency treatment, having been transferred there from the East Surrey Hospital, Redhill. While receiving an exceptional level of inpatient care from the trauma team, it provided us with a stark reminder of the mismatch between the quality of care skilled staff are able to achieve when using the latest equipment and the inferior facilities provided in your St James' Wing. Much better facilities would help the trauma team to carry out its complex surgical procedures and the processes of recovery through complicated inpatient and outpatient care even more successfully.

As you are the chief transformation officer, we are wondering if your trust board might consider building a new major trauma centre at St George's. This could demonstrate how to make a difference to your work at St George's and in a wider context, be an exemplar for the improvement of the NHS building environment. This would be planned to respond to the skills of your trauma team and relieve it from being embedded In the St James' Wing.

A new St George's Major Trauma Centre, serving its extensive catchment area of South West London, Surrey, and parts of East and West Sussex, could provide a new stand alone, fully self-sufficient facility with up to 64 inpatient rooms (beds) to replace the 54 beds on H and G Wards. It would also contain a new A&E, radiology, theatre, consulting examination suites and support facilities and be seen to be a beacon of hope for St George's and the NHS (our brochure illustrates what this might look like). A new state-of-the-art centre could also go some way towards sorting out the appalling congestion and the stressful and disorientating experience for patients accessing the current hospital facilities.

If you could find time to read our brochure, you will see that our proposals follow on from our participation in central government policy and guidance over many years. We are not looking for work as we are happily retired. We just wish that at least one trust could use the wealth of existing data to show how to create a new smaller hospital that could be assembled quickly, be affordable within a fixed capital cost (not to exceed 10,000 sq. metres in size) and have more relevance to the way clinical teams will need to operate in the future. It should also be uncomplicated, understandable, flexible and intensively used. When, over time, it reaches its sell-by date and becomes inflexible and obstructive, it should be able to be easily decommissioned, deconstructed, and replaced without fuss.

LB = DECORATOR/PATIENT

Is St George's up for a challenge such as this? It would seem to us that a new stand-alone major trauma centre, as outlined above, might be a perfect fit with the priorities in your current five-year strategy (2019-2024). Also, where better than at St George's to showcase to the wider NHS how the right kind of new, stand-alone, smaller, smarter, hospital could be provided in many parts of the country to prioritise the gaps in provision rather than repeating the mistake of over-investing in new unaffordable large hospitals in very few locations. We have had decades to understand, in project after project, that large hospitals have always cost more than they should, are never delivered on time, become obsolete too soon and unmanageable for far too long.

We are sending a copy of this email with a hard copy of our brochure to your home address in case you are working from home during this latest lockdown. It might take a little longer to reach you by post!

Kind regards

29th January 2021

Email to Dear Chief Transformation Officer from LB and RG

Dear James

Thank you for making time to phone us last Friday about the issues you, your team, and the trust board have had to wrestle with over the last three years or so. Clearly it is a massive task to transform St George's, having completed projects like the Moorfields Suite, to find solutions to improve other less productive services/specialties and provide new services in such a complex, large, teaching hospital.

At the same time, you are having to deal with major Infrastructure problems, backlog maintenance deficits and a need to rationalise the shared estate with its many aging obsolete buildings obstructing the transformation process. These, until demolished, sit on land that might be sold off or developed to benefit the hospital.

If all this is not enough, St George's has had to respond to the demands of Covid-19, revamping the hospital to safeguard patients and staff, doubling the number of intensive care beds and still keeping non-Coronavirus specialties like the major trauma centre up and running.

As said on Friday, thankfully we are retired and do not have to deal with the problems presented by a large failing teaching hospital such as yours which, as we know from our own recent experience of your inpatient facilities, is able to provide an exceptional level of patient care against the odds. It was only after needing the service provided by your major trauma centre that we thought to send you our email of 19th January with our brochure and to dare ask if you would consider building your highly skilled trauma team a purpose-built, stand-alone trauma centre.

From our brochure, you will have seen that we set out to suggest an alternative to the building of new large hospitals given the dramatic changes the country faces following the pandemic. After many decades of building large hospitals and giving ourselves insurmountable long-term problems, we think smaller hospitals might be the answer to the problem of updating and matching the future demands of the NHS.

We also suggested in our brochure that we should only look at transforming existing large hospitals when there is space on site to build a smaller, stand-alone hospital. The idea being that the design of a new smaller hospital would not only take on board lessons learnt from the upheaval caused by the pandemic but also stand alone, uncontaminated, by

LB = DECORATOR/PATIENT

inappropriate operational policies of the existing hospital. What to do with empty parts of the existing hospital could be resolved when the new hospital is near to up and running and, when it is clearer, whether to refurbish, or more sensibly, to close vacated premises.

It was with these thoughts in mind that we wondered whether a new major trauma centre might be built on your 'Visitor 1' car park site, having demolished the no longer used and boarded up Claire House and Bronte House – a perfect, substantial site in a prominent position. A new access road directly into this site might be formed from a new roundabout at the junction of Blackshaw Road and Muybury Street for emergency ambulances and to serve the new stand-alone major trauma centre (perhaps this site is one of those allocated for housing?).

Imagine turning off Tooting High Street into Blackshaw Road, arriving at a newly constructed roundabout, looking across and up at a new, imposing, inspirational, stand-alone, smart, major trauma centre. This could be the jewel in the crown of a transformed St George's, able to demonstrate to a recovering NHS that all is alive and well. It should look more like an impressive and sophisticated piece of well-designed/engineered hospital equipment rather than a traditional run-of-the-mill hospital building, allowing patients, visitors, and staff to approach it with renewed confidence about what this new type of facility might deliver. Ho-hum, how easy to dream and fantasize!

Following your call, we decided to rehearse our thoughts again in this email to understand our fantasy in relation to your real-world hospital and its pressing challenges. We are not expecting you to reply to this email as thankfully you have given us more time than we deserve. We appreciate that you see your major trauma centre becoming part of a comprehensive refurbishment to provide an emergency floor for a range of specialties, which is altogether a different concept.

Best wishes for your task of transforming St George's

Kind Regards

29th January 2021

Email to LB and RG from Chief Transformation Officer

Thanks, both – good 'rehearsing' – I'm hoping to be able to invite you to see around our new emergency floor facility in a few years' time.

Best wishes

James

Mysteriously, within the year, James' photo was removed from the hospital notice board. When enquiring about what had happened to James at the Orthoplastic clinic, one of the consultants said he had been transformed!

Chapter 6
"We will build 40 New Hospitals"

One of the earliest political promises made in 2020 when the nation was totally preoccupied with Covid was that funding would be allocated to provide the NHS with 40 new hospitals.[5] Plans to build a new 300-bed hospital in Sutton, Surrey, were at an advanced stage and arrangements for a public consultation were in-hand. The consultation period was due to close on 1st April 2020 during the first Covid lockdown. The

---

[5] Some sources estimate that another 5000 beds should be provided to help to fix the NHS. If the NHS can begin to train up more staff able to operate highly sophisticated new hospitals and plug the current exodus of experienced staff, it maybe will not need all these new beds – especially if 20 or so of the right kind of new hospitals are provided quickly. The NHS can then sort out the immediate demand. The issue surely is about movement, throughput, turnover, and improving outcomes, not just about bed numbers. On 7th January during the PM's first interview in 2023 he mentioned to Laura Kuenssberg initiatives such as the setting up of a national 'discharge fund', 'virtual wards' to accommodate patients not needing hospital care, and 'ambulance triage' to deal with some people at home to stem the flow of A&E arrivals. Initiatives such as these should not prevent getting on with the urgent provision of new-style smaller 2020s hospitals described above. If enough of these were to be built, they would have an immediate impact on all other initiatives.

LB = DECORATOR/PATIENT

local NHS was allocated £500 million to invest in hospital buildings subject to this consultation.

As early as March 2020, it was looking like a proposal to build a new 300-bed hospital in Sutton based on what went before Covid might not be the best solution for the 2020s. Does it make any sense to build an old-style district general hospital, even if you call it a 'specialist emergency care hospital' in new speak, when it was becoming obvious that nucleus hospitals and other large hospitals were no longer the answer for the NHS. Everyone could see how hospitals were struggling to deal with the Covid pandemic when needing to convert wards to quadruple the number of intensive care and high-dependency beds. So much so, it was decided – wrongly – to provide never-to-be-used additional beds in open plan wards in instant temporary Nightingale hospitals – what a nightmare. Florence would have turned in her grave.

What is now clear at last is that wards with large multi-bed bays are not only unpleasant but also unmanageable. If one ever did need convincing that single rooms with ensuite toilets and showers should be the new norm it certainly should be obvious after Covid that this must be the way forward. All patients should be allowed privacy, dignity, and respect when admitted for inpatient care, especially as it is, nowadays, likely to be for a serious life-changing or life-threatening condition, if not Covid. Even if it is not as a trauma or acute admission, but to give birth or to receive care for a chronic medical or geriatric condition, surely a patient deserves to be nursed or cared for in a single room.

Having experienced Covid at its worst, it does not make sense to spend £500 million on one local NHS to build a 300-bed hospital. Less money would be better spent on new, easy, smart, smaller 2020s hospitals. Large hospitals are too big to handle. They take forever to plan and build and require updating on completion. When they facilitate bad practice, it is not easily changed and because of its size and complexity, almost impossible to replace.

From now on no hospital building should be regarded as long-life. New smaller 2020s hospitals could stand alone uncontaminated by what is going on around them if they must be built on an existing hospital site. They should be affordable, uncomplicated, understandable, flexible, intensively used, inspiring beacons of hope and promise. They should have less than 100 beds and most of these should be in single bedrooms with ensuites. These smaller hospitals should be complete and self-sufficient with all facilities in place, including emergency admissions, X-ray, theatres, recovery, outpatients and rehabilitation. They would be small enough for patients, visitors, and staff to be informed about what is going on within the building and promote team working with no hiding places. These smaller dynamic hospitals might look less like a hospital, with an ambience providing a more therapeutic and supportive environment. This could be instrumental in helping all users to feel informed, reassured, and positive about what is on offer.

The conclusion of the public consultation in April 2020 was that the local NHS should build a 300-bed hospital in Sutton. The £500 million allocation was confirmed.

LB = DECORATOR/PATIENT

Having time on their hands during the first lockdown, it seemed reasonable for two residents served by this local NHS to draw attention to their doubts and to respond to this public consultation. Particularly so because these two residents had access to much of the policy and health building documentation produced over many decades. Not only was there time for doubts to be put forward about the proposed new hospital but there was time to produce a brochure setting out alternatives. This illustrated brochure showed how a new, easy, fast, smart, smaller hospital might look but it did not strike the right chord at the time. It has always been too difficult to divert the NHS from its set ways, even when Covid is in town.

Maybe a realisation that to continue to build inefficient, large hospitals is not in the interest of the NHS will only come about after a few mega hospitals have been constructed.

These will then confirm what we already know – that they can facilitate bad practice, which is not easily changed. Large hospitals can be seen to be too much for patients and staff to comprehend when faced with a maze of rooms and corridors, which misinform, disorientate, and increase dependency. Unfortunately, some members of a lobby group called Architects for Health promote the building of European super hospitals.

Who knows whether the 40 new hospitals promised will fix the NHS and restore the health of the Nation? However, we should avoid building European super hospitals and large hospitals.

Chapter 7
Dear Clare and Dear District Council

This chapter is included to show that responding to a call to participate in a public consultation for whatever reason is a kind of self-harm. You know when you start to become involved that your comments, if different to what is wanted, will probably end up in an independent analysis report appendix highlighting alternative suggestions, or binned without acknowledgement. This is no matter who you are or where you have been all your life. Knowing that this is life's rich pattern helps you to be persistent to get not very far – as this book shows. Persistence is easier when you are at home for the Covid-19 lockdown, or holed up for a couple of years on your back with your leg elevated. Somehow, you are always up and ready to email those people not wanting to hear from you – perhaps rightly but surely someone should bother?

So here are another couple of emails to confirm that no one really wants to hear from you. This is to do with another proposal from NHS South West London to put a new renal unit at St George's as part of its transformation.

LB = DECORATOR/PATIENT

26th October 2021

Email to Dear Clare from LB

[Dear Clare is the Consultation and Engagement lead at SWLNHS]

Dear Clare

Thank you for keeping me informed.

I do not have a problem with the engagement plan. As claimed it is robust. Clearly the response from patients and staff has confirmed a real belief that change is essential. Engagement has attracted keen support for the preferred option to provide a new joint renal centre at St George's to replace failing facilities at both St George's and St Helier hospitals. It is now well understood that existing renal facilities at both these hospitals have served their purpose well but are now obstructing service development.

My interest is in understanding whether proposals can ever match expectations and levels of support shown in the engagement report and analysis when the new renal centre is built at St George's.

Alternative sites within the wider catchment area to those at St George's, St Helier and the new hospital at Sutton should have been part of the consultation process. This might have encouraged stakeholders and local authorities outside South West London in the wider catchment area to engage with the consultations and fully participate in the provision of dispersed but well connected local NHS services.

Mole Valley District Council is one of several district councils within the catchment area of the current renal service. It has recently published for consultation it's new draft local plan. All district councils have had to undertake exercises to identify sites available for development primarily for housing. Mole Valley has selected two sites in Dorking for development (ref Policy DS23: Pixham End Southern Parcel on the A24 and DS24: Sondes Place Farm on the A25). I think both would be ideal for a new state-of-the-art, self-sufficient, joint renal centre and theatres for a radically different dispersed renal service serving South West London, Surrey and East and West Sussex. Either of these sites might be used to demonstrate how new NHS facilities might break the mould in moving off long-established but failing hospital sites which are now known to be in the wrong place for future service provision.

Before the die is cast, perhaps your business case might explore the notion of using smaller alternative sites in the right location for key hospital specialties like renal services. This just might indicate cost benefits in providing better-dispersed services. It could also showcase how the right buildings in the right place could enhance service performance to benefit patients throughout the NHS.

Best wishes

LB

1st November 2021

Email from Dear Clare to LB

Dear LB

Thank you for taking the time to share your views on the recent engagement regarding improvements to kidney care.

You may have seen that questions were raised during the engagement regarding more detail on the rationale of choosing St George's as the site for the proposed specialist renal unit. This will be addressed on the decision-making business case.

Thank you again for your interest.

Clare

LB = DECORATOR/PATIENT

1st November 2021

Email to N&N from LB

[N had a kidney transplant 28 years ago at St Helier Hospital (a significant success)[6]]

Dear N&N

Please see latest. I am not sure how long I will keep this up as the jargon sends me to sleep!

Uncle xx

7th November 2021

Email to District Council from LB & RG

Dear Sir/madam

Re: new Draft Local Plan (Regulation 19)

Thank you for the opportunity to comment on your new draft local plan. We are pleased to note that this is much improved and that the green belt 'take' has been significantly reduced. Also, that the brownfield allocation is now greater than the loss of green belt. It will be interesting to see what the planning inspector makes of the proposed reduction in the housing target which we fully support in order to protect

---

[6] Time waits for no one!. N&N = Niece (Beryl) & Nil (nephew-in-law - Kieran). Kieran died in the Intensive Care Unit at St Helier Hospital on 20th April 2023.

Kieran used with joy his gift of 28 years of life. He was the perfect advert for an outstanding renal service provided by the NHS. Kieran, niece Beryl and the renal service staff walked hand in hand into the unknown for many years. Together they were to witness the growth in expertise in renal care which now clearly needs something different from the general hospital facilities provided today at St Helier Hospital. Kieran will be missed by so many.

the character of Mole Valley's great landscape value around and between its towns and villages.

On looking again at the proposed development sites, it occurs to us that some of these would be suitable for mixed developments or non-housing projects, especially the larger sites near town centres. Also, we are wondering if more could be done to promote development opportunities for community projects that would benefit from being located near town centres but still connected with areas of outstanding natural beauty, i.e. educational and recreational facilities and health and social care buildings using, for example, the two outstanding sites in Dorking on the A24 (Policy DS23: Pixham End) and the A25 (Policy D524: Sondes Place) now earmarked for what could be a sympathetic expansion of a remarkable market town rather than more suburbs of little boxes all in a row as around Horsham.

The pandemic has caused a change in working practices including working from home and this could lead to a dispersal of services that previously were likely to be more centralised. For example, 95 percent of local NHS renal services are community-based due to significant changes like home dialysis with less reliance on major hospital sites. New renal services might be located to be accessible and therapeutic on one or two of these sites using your planning constraints listed with each site helping to safeguard and sympathetically relate developments to some of the adjacent open spaces, views, and local characteristics of these sites. A mix of building types would help vary the densities of housing-only developments and could also reinvigorate the local economy. Perhaps Mole Valley could find a way of encouraging collaboration by sharing the local plan with non-local authority services like the NHS.

Subject to the above consideration re-mixed and non-housing developments, we believe the new local plan is an appropriate strategy taking into account reasonable alternatives and is based on proportionate evidence. Mole Valley District Council, across generations with the help of its active community, has always found ways to safeguard its areas of outstanding natural beauty and to achieve a balance when facing demands and challenges for redevelopment imposed on it by central government. The planning inspector should fully endorse its efforts to comply but accept that the district council is best placed to continue to protect its countryside and heritage, making Mole Valley one of the best places to live in our overdeveloped country.

RG & LB

As of January 2023, the district council's draft local plan is in limbo until the government reviews its policy for the green belt. Speculation is that both these sites will be used to provide essential housing and not a non-essential, dispersed, accessible and ground-breaking renal centre. Developer's housing plans are being circulated in advance to gauge public opinion before a formal planning application is made to test the water – whenever!

So, another not so bright idea bites the dust!

Chapter 8

Dear Mr Chairman - 2

Chapter 4 left the issue of written evidence to the chairman of the Select Committee open and subject to whether this was worth the effort and could be compiled in time... it was!

EVIDENCE TO THE HEALTH AND SOCIAL CARE COMMITTEE

It has been over a year since we forwarded to your committee a hard copy of our brochure[7] on 29th May 2020. In our brochure, we attempted to paint a picture of what a new, smaller, 2020 hospital might look like as a more affordable and quicker alternative to the kind of large-scale provision being proposed for Sutton, Surrey,

---

[7] Our brochure, *New, Easy, Fast, Smart, Smaller 2020 Hospitals to improve the NHS – after Covid-19*. Sent in hard copy to HSSC on 29th May 2020. It was subsequently circulated by your office in a digital format on 4th July 2020. This brochure was compiled during the first Coronavirus lockdown by two former employees of the Department of Health, having had access to much of the policy and health building documentation produced over many years to guide the NHS. It was thought that following Covid-19 there would be less money to invest in the replacement of the existing stock of NHS out-of-date, inflexible buildings that are no longer suitable for treating patients to modern healthcare standards.

and elsewhere. We anticipated that lessons learnt from the pandemic would expose the inadequacy of the tortuous planning processes, traditional ward and hospital layouts and highlight an urgent need to invest in new, smaller, more efficient facilities initially for trauma and elective services.

All over the country, there is a mismatch between the quality of care skilled staff are expected to achieve using the latest equipment in the worst kind of facilities. Surgical teams urgently need an opportunity to carry out complex surgical procedures and the processes for recovery in facilities designed to reflect lessons learnt from the pandemic.

Prior to the pandemic, efforts were being made in numerous localities to save, recover, maintain, and grow existing hospitals. Large teams were planning for change to radically update or replace failing hospitals. They often produced five-year plans to implement – but here lies the problem. The pandemic has rendered such long-term plans invalid, unaffordable, and unfit for purpose.

Surely now gone are the days of long-term planning cycles and public consultations leading to gradual and begrudging ways to improve redundant hospitals or to the provision of monolithic, inflexible new hospitals. These are guaranteed to remain or become a burden for decades. Covid-19 demands that we urgently change this mind set.

We believe we are approaching a time when realistically the provision of new hospitals has to be limited by capping capital allocations for all local NHS projects. This should be seen as a positive policy. A way to achieve this would be to inform local NHSs that they can bid to build a new, smaller 2020s trauma or elective hospital of up to 10,000 sq. m. if they can demonstrate that this would foster a radical new approach to their service provision, including, if possible, at an alternative location to the existing hospital. Existing hospitals were probably built in the right place for the 1900s but are most likely to be in the wrong place for the 2020s. A strategy providing a network of smaller hospitals would make land acquisition easier.

There is just not enough capacity in the NHS to deal with the current backlog in the short- and medium-term, so a rapid construction programme should always be a condition of funding. We are imagining the production of brand-new, smaller hospitals to kick-start a revitalised hospital construction programme. Stockpiles of data and guidance exist to inform how new, smaller hospitals might be planned, designed and commissioned in the 2020s. Example solutions used in our brochure were based on this wealth of information and which suggest how (A) a trauma centre and (B) an elective centre might be planned to create a new, smaller 2020s hospital within a 10,000 sq.m allocation. What is needed now is someone to sanction the construction of new, smaller hospital prototypes. An enthusiastic NHS team could be commissioned to plan, design, help arrange manufacture and, when fully operational, monitor and compare performance.

LB = DECORATOR/PATIENT

The pandemic has shown that we can learn to move quickly to provide the NHS with equipment and temporary facilities staff demanded for their own hospitals (they did not want to use those over-sized, wasteful and nightmarish Nightingale hospitals). It has also shown that new and better facilities are urgently required to tackle the waiting lists that are a consequence of the pandemic and that these should build in measures to contain Covid-19 surges.

To summarise, a new smaller hospital in the right location should probably be sited away from, but used in conjunction with, an existing hospital, be assembled quickly, be affordable within a fixed capital cost (up to 10,000 sq. m. in size), and have more relevance to the way surgical teams will have to work in the future. It should also be uncomplicated, patient friendly, therapeutic, flexible, and intensively used.

Now is the time to showcase how adaptable, new, smaller hospitals can be provided quickly to replace our many failing hospitals. These would lift morale, renew confidence, and house and promote even better services throughout the NHS. The primary aim should be to demonstrate that the NHS will require less beds, not more, through improved performances in the right kind of facilities in the aftermath of this life changing pandemic.

If your committee really is interested in recognising how much the NHS estate and existing hospital buildings are straightjacketing innovation as services need to evolve to meet emerging challenges, here is a tentative road map:

1. DHSC to appoint a control team to set up parameters for a network of new, smaller 2020s hospitals and project manage the provision and evaluation of the first wave.
2. Organise an open invitation to local NHSs with a five-year plan, asking them to put their plans on the back burner and, instead, apply to be selected to build a new, smaller 2020s trauma or elective hospital.
3. Set up a selection process for a first wave network focussing on the following: the applicant's surgical team's performance and their proposals to deal with waiting lists; management and staff cohesion; an ability to show how they might operate the new facility; their ways and means of demonstrating a better performance from new facilities; availability of a potential site and its location; how each local NHS is ready to move quickly to provide a new facility, and, on completion, how the evacuation of existing hospital accommodation might be used to improve other priority services including long Covid.
4. Completion, commissioning and a fully operational service should be documented as a case study for a second wave.
5. Each new smaller hospital should be evaluated to report on performance.

We are looking for no more than an indication that some of our suggestions might be relevant to a rebuilt

NHS, taking account of Covid-19 and the need for an increased capacity to deal with the backlog. Also, we are looking for signs that your committee is taking seriously a need to build the right kind of hospitals to support the future work of the NHS and care services. Buildings cannot put more staff in place to deal with the backlog but they can give staff within the NHS better facilities to help improve and increase performances.

LB and RG

> *3rd September 2021*
>
> *Email to LB from No reply@Parliament*
>
> *Dear LB and RG*
>
> *Thank you for submitting written evidence to the Health and Social Care Committee's inquiry, 'clearing the backlog caused by the pandemic.'*
>
> *We have received your submission made on 03/09/2021 15:55:1, and we are processing it.*
>
> *We will send you a further notification when your evidence has been accepted as a submission and published on the committee's website...*
>
> *Thank you for your interest in our work.*

Around this time, details about another project being planned for South West London, Surrey and East and West Sussex were released for public consultation. This proposal was to replace and combine the two renal units at St George's and St Helier with a preference for it to be sited at St George's (Teaching) Hospital.

Not only did it make sense to respond to the public consultation but it also felt appropriate to email the Health and Social Care Select Committee – again!

2nd November 2021

Email to Health and Social Care Committee from L B

Dear Health and Social Care Committee

Given that I have not heard further following my submission of written evidence on 03/09/2021, I assume there is little interest from your committee in providing smaller hospital units quickly as a means of clearing the backlog caused by the pandemic.

Perhaps this is not surprising given that issues raised by others in their written evidence will be concerned with staffing numbers, recruitment and training. However, I am relieved to see that Professor Stephen Powis, when giving evidence to your committee, dared discuss building design-related ideas for hospitals of the future. His promotion of single rooms at last brought to the fore the connection between the right kind of health care buildings and an improved performance in outcomes. In dealing with the massive backlog and the disruption caused by the pandemic, the NHS's inadequate stock of health care buildings must be seen as a major obstacle because many facilities are known to need replacing.

If someone on your committee has the time and inclination to read further into the unbelievable processes now laboured over in the NHS to replace failing hospitals with facilities which should aid rather than hinder service development, I am forwarding separately recent emails and links between me and the South West London NHS renal team. I was staggered to see that they were proposing to build a new renal centre to serve South West London, Surrey and East

LB = DECORATOR/PATIENT

and West Sussex at St George's Hospital, Tooting, a large, congested teaching hospital with a track record of failure. Surely a recognition that the existing facilities at St George's and St Helier hospitals must be replaced with a new joint renal centre should be seen as a chance to try something different for a renal service where 95 percent of the service has evolved to become dispersed across a very large catchment area.

Perhaps this decision will be reviewed by South West London NHS and the renal team at the business case stage to clarify the choice of location. To me, it seems that the only reason to locate a joint renal centre at St George's is to safeguard the ongoing long-term project to transform this large failing hospital which surely should end up being reduced rather than expanded in size. As a consequence of the pandemic, we should now be looking to see if there are better ways to match future health care facilities with potentially progressive, localised specialist services and be less inclined to revamp and expand large hospitals like St George's just because it has always been there. The transformation of a long-term failing teaching hospital into a mega hospital will not change it from being in a congested part of South West London on a crowded, badly serviced and overdeveloped site shared with a large university medical school that is also competing for space.

As suggested in our previous exchanges, I believe urgent consideration should be given to providing a network of affordable, new, easy, fast, smart, smaller, standalone trauma and elective care hospital units if we really do want to be effective in clearing the backlog caused by the pandemic. Similarly, smaller hospitals could also be used for other much-needed specialities like the renal centre now being considered by the South West London renal team in order for it to be located where it can best serve its catchment area. If only...!

Best wishes for your inquiry.

LB

Date: Jan 10, 2022 12:31:16 PM

Subject: Re: Clearing the backlog caused by the pandemic

Dear Mr LB

Can I firstly apologise for taking so long to get back to you. We receive a large amount of correspondence through the committee inbox and it can take some time to get through it all.

Thank you for submitting evidence to our inquiry. It was helpful as we came to draft our report on our inquiry into 'Clearing the backlog caused by the pandemic'.

I hope you will have noticed that we have published our report this week. If you have not, here is a link for you to read the report: https://committees.parliment.uk/publications/8352/documents/85020/default/

You will also likely be aware of the surgical hub model being piloted throughout the NHS in England as means of clearing the backlog. However, the issues of resource allocation in healthcare, as you make clear, is complex. For your specific example, I would suggest that you raise this issue directly with your own MP as it is a local issue.

Best wishes

Chair, Health and Social Care Committee

House of Commons I London I SW1A PAA

Chapter 9

Dear Susan and Dear Mr Consultant

Emails to Dear Susan continued over a long period. These were often used to seek help and advice when things appeared not to be working, for example:

16th December 2021

Email to Dear Susan from decorator/patient

Dear Susan

As you may know, I was sent a brief text message cancelling my appointment to attend the trauma and orthopaedic outpatient clinic today – the 16th December.

Without an explanation, I assume that NHS resources have been actioned to deal with the pandemic, the Omicron variant, a possible surge in bed numbers, and the recently announced end of year target to booster jab all willing sections of the population.

Unfortunately, it seems that clearing the massive backlog caused by the pandemic has again had to take a backseat. Also, trauma patients like me, admitted as emergencies since the first lockdown via A&E, seem now to be becoming part of the ever increasing backlog.

With your support, I have been attending St George's for over a year now. I have had six operations under full anaesthetic and 13 visits to the outpatients clinic. Mr Consultant informed me on my last visit four weeks ago that I have a 50:50 chance of saving or losing my leg below my right knee. St George's and Mr Consultant have skilfully invested heavily in my recovery with still much to do!

Can someone please tell me if it makes sense to cancel or withdraw my orthopaedic supervision until after Christmas? At this crucial point in my treatment I would like to know how I can reduce the odds on recovering the use of my leg without attending outpatients!

It makes sense for the country to deal with the pandemic but for me it certainly does not make sense to waste a whole year's effort on saving my leg because St George's cannot manage an immunisation programme and its consequences, and also maintain its usual hospital services at the same time. Is there no one who can see that the ever-increasing backlog could lead to a health care crisis that could outstrip the pandemic?

Sorry to keep using you as a conduit – perhaps Mr Consultant and the trauma team might be interested to see how these decisions are affecting at least one of its patients.

Best wishes and kind regards to you and Mr Consultant

LB

Within two hours, decorator/patient received a telephone call from St George's reinstating the appointment the same day at 4pm.

Other emails sent to Dear Susan were sent with Mr Consultant in mind to thank him and to try to give something back to the trauma team.

For new, easy, smart, smaller 2020s hospitals to be seen to be an answer to the crisis facing the NHS, it would make sense to build one to test the water. Chapter 5 gives an insight into why this was not possible at St George's even though it has a specialist major trauma team. This trauma team does not appear to have the facilities needed to completely control its own performance and patient outcomes. So, the decorator/patient/retired architect had another go at making the case!

16th February 2022

Email to Dear Susan from decorator/patient

Dear Susan

Would you please forward the email below to Mr Consultant?

Also, I would like to thank you for your patience when dealing with my demanding emails and for pointing me in the right direction in a timely manner.

Best wishes

LB

Dear Mr Consultant

It was good to hear your encouraging news about my progress at the outpatient appointment on 20th January 2022 – thank you to you, your senior registrars, and team for my care and attention over many months.

Perhaps, as a retired architect who specialized in the design of hospitals, I needed to endure late-in-life hospitalization at St George's to remind myself how skilled NHS staff are expected to work miracles in outdated hospital buildings. You may be interested to see

LB = DECORATOR/PATIENT

the following feedback from one of your patients with time on his hands!

As a consequence of the arrival of Covid-19 in early 2020 and my subsequent admission as a trauma patient to St George's Hospital in November 2020, I became convinced that a different approach to the design of hospital buildings is needed. So convinced that in January 2021, my wife, Rosemary, a retired health administrator, and I asked the director of transformation at St George's to try something different from the proposals in his five-year plan and to consider building a stand-alone major trauma centre, befitting the service and skills of the St George's trauma and orthopaedics team. This perhaps was a bit cheeky but seemed worth a try in desperate times.

This could have provided a fresh beginning to replace the 54 orthopaedic beds in H and G Wards which are too chaotic and crowded, mostly in multi-bed bays (and worse still, those orthopaedic beds randomly allocated in a 'green' V Ward). The idea being that new trauma centre would give the trauma team full control of its own exclusive facility consisting of suites for emergency admissions, radiology, theatres, rehabilitation, outpatients, administration, and 64 beds, mainly in single-bed rooms. An improved turnover justifying the expense.

We thought this might be done quickly to show the NHS a new way forward. Sadly, this was not possible. Not unreasonably – it is difficult to abandon long-term plans to transform a large failing hospital like St George's. Plans began to take shape in 2017 before the pandemic and are likely take another three or four years to complete. However, with Covid-19 hitting the fan, experiences have shown a need to do things differently. Long-term plans are no longer an appropriate response. Neither is the temptation to panic buy temporary accommodation (like the unused Nightingale hospitals or similar!).

In tandem with our many visits to St George's over the past 14 months, Rosemary and I have also been trying to convince the parliamentary Health and Social Care Select Committee that the design of new hospitals could have a bearing on how the NHS might recover from its own trauma, cope with the vaccine-shackled virus from now on, and get to grips with clearing the massive backlog caused by the pandemic. Again, not unreasonably, interest was restrained perhaps because it has been an exceptionally busy time for the HSCC or because resource allocation in healthcare is too complex. At least our 'written evidence' was attached to the HSCC's inquiry report, 'Clearing the backlog caused by the pandemic', published in January 2022. The committee chose not to run with our suggestion that it should be possible for the NHS to build its way out of its problems by urgently building only additional new smaller trauma and elective care hospitals. However, it did encourage the setting up of surgical hubs for elective care without recommending the kind of facilities needed. We argued that if and when new trauma and elective care centres became operational, existing hospitals, where salvageable, might then be recalibrated for other priority specialties including long Covid.

Plan 1 attached illustrates how a fantasy, standalone, all-singing and dancing Trauma Centre A might look. This is shown alongside a fantasy Elective Care Centre B.

We now see our suggestions as a missed opportunity especially knowing that construction of a new major trauma centre at St George's could have been well underway by now if started soon after January 2021! However, these fantasy illustrations might provide you with a useful reference if you ever find yourself involved in planning a major trauma centre at some point in the future or as a teaching aid to promote discussion. We think we have learnt that trauma teams need facilities that help

LB = DECORATOR/PATIENT

improve performance, assist in reducing recovery times, and give patients a better deal when facing a life- or limb-threatening trauma. Also, we think we are clearer about what a surgical hub for elective care might need to look like.

There you have it – I pass these thoughts on to you with thanks for handling my recovery from my self-inflicted trauma. Having attempted to give the NHS something back in return, I now feel that I can limp off into the sunset!

Kind regards

LB

It was hardly surprising that this got no reaction from Mr Consultant. You only need to visit the Orthoplastic clinic's crammed waiting room to see that there is more than enough to do there and in the operating theatres too! All staff are so incredibly busy and it is difficult for them to draw breath let alone think about what might be done to change things.

Sometime later decorator/patient emailed Dear Susan again – this time to provide Mr Consultant with feedback about the service provided to him by the St George's Hospital major trauma team and others. It was thought that this might be of more interest to Mr Consultant than the 'pigs might fly' canvassing for a new trauma centre.

23rd May 2022

Email to Dear Susan from decorator/patient

Dear Susan

Hope this finds you well – one final favour please?

I would appreciate it if you could forward this to Mr Consultant. It is a last word from one of his patients who has had time to tell!

Best wishes

LB

Dear Mr Consultant

A patient with a view! (Further to my email of 16/2/22)

It was good to see you at your clinic on 5th May. These clinics are always very business-like and brief without feeling rushed (and sometimes very enjoyable) but leave little time for reflection. You therefore may be interested in this summary of notes made about my recovery over a 17-month period.

Following my fall from grace on 26th November 2020, I have attended St George's for five operations under full anaesthetic (following a first at the East Surrey Hospital). I have had three stopovers as an inpatient where the longest period was for ten days. I have experienced good orthopaedic inpatient care on H Ward despite its outdated facilities and nursing care unfamiliar with the needs of orthopaedic patients on an equally out dated 'green' V Ward. I have also attended 16 outpatient clinics (has anyone ever wondered how patients and escorts are able to be beamed down into your clinic on time for appointments?) and ten visits to a very efficient X-ray department. All of this was as a passive patient, mostly prone with my leg elevated and adorned with plaster casts, a Prof Ilizarov external fixator (for four months) or a surgical boot/air walker (for most of the time). I was unfortunate that my fall coincided with the pandemic but I will always remain grateful that somehow your trauma team, well supported by theatre staff and the X-ray department, remained active through all this chaos.

It has not been easy for me to achieve continuity of care living in Dorking – part of the trauma team's outreach catchment extending from St George's as far as Surrey and East and West Sussex. My GP practice has not been available for face-to-face support throughout most of my recovery period and local physiotherapy services closed because of Covid until April 2021. From then on, GP referrals for physiotherapy have been hindered by further surgery at St George's or more recently a reluctance by physiotherapists to provide a service from Dorking Hospital without access to my medical records. Fortunately, the district nursing service kept going during the pandemic's second lockdown and through the early phase of my recovery. This provided me with beyond-the-call-of-duty home visits from December 2020, often two times a week, to change incision and open wound dressings and to keep on top of infections. Eventually the GP practice nurses were able to take over from the district nurses in September 2021 when they provided me with a continuing monitoring service until February this year. The district nurses and the GP nurses were given occasional support from your team when asked because there was minimal GP backup.

Over 17 months there have been moments when it was unclear whether my right ankle would ever recover. Perhaps not surprisingly ups and downs along the path to recovery have at times been traumatic. As recently as November 2021, I was given only a 50:50 chance that my *right leg below the knee could be saved following the removal of the external fixator. Those odds improved in December 2021 to 65:35, in January 2022 to 80:20, in March to 90:10, and finally 95:5 on 5th May. The relatively recent sprint to achieve walking-stick-aided mobility is rewarding but baffling!*

It now seems from the March X-rays that the four fractures are at last beginning to knit together. An ongoing concern has been how long it has taken to completely heal the incision wound along the shin. Even now, a small area needs attention although seemingly not infected. The soft tissue around my ankle is recovering well with periodic swelling and redness – thankfully I am experiencing little pain.

Physiotherapy is still a thorny issue and at the moment it is difficult to know whether or not it could ever help my recovery. I am still unsure if I should be wearing the air walker for supported mobility. When I am out and about without the air walker, using an NHS issue walking stick, or at home without either the air walker or the walking stick, the ankle seems to be getting stronger. I am no longer wearing the air walker during the night following discussion at your clinic on 17th March this year. It is still hard to judge whether to do without the air walker when walking longer distances, undertaking physical activities like watering the garden, or when attending appointments and social events. Since the 5th May, I have tried to do without it as wearing the air walker seems to distort my ankle and restrict progress.

As you know, I have always had a long-term target to get to Greece, having booked my flight for 24th May well in advance. My aim has always been to be able to swim to the harbour wall from the town beach at my holiday destination! So, I will soon see just what is possible with or *without the air walker although, as advised, I will probably wear it for the journey.*

The most difficult part of being a trauma patient, apart from a total dependence on my wife, family, and friends, is the time it takes to recover, accompanied by a gradual loss of general physical fitness. I have had to take time out from the way I lived my previous life to wait for the healing process to occur. I am wondering if more might be done to expose patients to a more comprehensive, rigorous, and accessible recovery programme where surgical and non-surgical specialist are coordinated, fully available, and informed. The waiting game for recovery is really demotivating. Is there no way of speeding things up for lower limb trauma patients or will they always have to wear a ball and chain of some description while waiting for nature to take its unnatural course – assisted by skilled corrective surgery when required? Maybe things were different before the pandemic but it does seem to me that a co-ordinated recovery programme might help produce a different outcome. For example, might the 'plastics' nurses at St George's have been better placed to treat my incisions and open wounds and provide infection control more successfully than the district nurses or the GP practice nurses? When making frequent visits to St George's for outpatient appointments, might it have been better to spend half a day or even a whole day at the hospital to tap into advice from all trauma team specialists? This might include follow-up appointments with orthopaedic/plastics nurses, physiotherapist, OTs, GPs, etc. to provide them with the responsibility to coordinate recovery with local services in the wider catchment area between regular visits to St George's – or is this just pure fantasy and only possible in an ideal NHS!

Your major trauma centre team knows full well how seriously restricted it is by the outdated facilities at

St George's and its reliance on hit-and-miss local services in its wider catchment area. Also, that this is likely to remain the case when the newly converted 'medical floor' becomes operational in 2024/25 because recovery is more than inspirational surgery.

You will know from my email to you of 16th February that I believe that the kind of facilities available to the NHS must affect clinical performance and recovery and that St George's needs a proper trauma centre. It also seems to me that outreach services from St George's to the trauma team's wider catchment area and collaboration with local services must be greatly improved.

I take my hat off to you and your surgical team for striving to help me keep my lower right leg and to make me mobile again against all the odds – it will be interesting to know if I can swim or sink in Greece!

Kind regards

LB

23rd May 2022

Email from Dear Susan to decorator/patient

Dear LB

Mr Consultant thanks you for your thoughts and feedback. He wishes you well for your swim.

Susan

Who else is likely to show some interest and, more to the point, want to do something to find a new approach to change things where it matters most – the new Secretary of State for Health and Social Care?

Chapter 10

The Great Escape – May 2022

The senior registrar who took over from Dear Zoe looked exactly like the kind of orthopaedic surgeon you would want to fix your trauma. Alistair is good-looking, blond, and built like a professional rugby player who could play the role of Biggles in a Hollywood movie. He was only lacking a half-decent bedside manner. At the clinic on 16th December 2021, he asked the decorator/patient what his expectations were for the foreseeable future. Sensing that a good year message might be forthcoming, the decorator/patient said he was expecting to be able to fly to Greece in May 2022, walk to sunbathe on a sandy beach, and swim to a nearby harbour wall. Alistair said that this was unlikely to happen. It was at this clinic that the odds were set at 65:35 in favour of saving the right leg below the knee.

Given that Alistair was the surgeon who removed Professor Ilizarov's external fixator on the 9th November 2021, who could argue?

Immediately, flights were booked for departure to Kalamata on 24th May 2022. So much would depend on what might happen over the next four to five months, with or without Alistair's encouragement!

There were to be another three clinic appointments before take-off. Progress, following the issue of a new surgical boot at the clinic on 16th December 2021, until the clinic on 20th January 2022, was slow but sure – it became possible to walk short distances around the garden like a teddy bear!

> 16th December 2021
>
> WhatsApp group from decorator/patient
>
> On my way home having shed the Chelsea-blue cast for a dull grey surgical boot. I've been told this is good news. Progress is a long haul at St George's but it seems from the smiles of the consultant and his registrar that the ankle is recovering. So, roll on Christmas with a spring in the step.
>
> 20th January 2022
>
> WhatsApp group from decorator/patient
>
> We have good cheer on Anna's birthday and encouragement from a cautious consultant and team... the odds are improving. It seems that the fractures are beginning to knit. This means I should start walking as is comfortable.

These WhatsApp messages are tailored for the family and to report on progress as instant news is now the name of the game – even more so when family visiting is restricted. More detailed feedback about the service provided by St George's is set out in a letter to Mr Consultant in Chapter 9.

17*th* March 2022

WhatsApp group from decorator/patient

We are just limping out of St George's – not for the last time. They want to review progress again two weeks before we leave for Greece in nine weeks' time to check that I am fit to swim to the harbour wall… I can now sleep without the dreaded boot… For the first time in 15 months the team seemed pleased with their work even though the leg is a funny shape.

It was becoming possible to get about and to start living life again by enjoying the occasional pub lunch. During April, progress was such that longer walks, sometimes without the boot, became more frequent, including a long-awaited visit to the dentist a short walk from Victoria Station. The dentist, who had thought his patient had passed away, made a ground-floor treatment room available. He found the teeth in good shape, was complimentary about the high standard of oral hygiene, but was very concerned about the state of the leg. Being Greek, he fully supported the need to escape to Greece but suggested avoiding a climb to the top of the Acropolis in Athens and every mountain in the Peloponnese.

On the 4th April, Whitstable was chosen for a first overnight stay away from the safety of home to test the water for the trip to Greece. In order to enjoy oysters and lobsters around the harbour you need to carefully select a seafront hotel only a short walk away. Margate was near enough to visit the new Tate with lift but the stepped approach to the entrance from the carpark, while fully appreciated as an architectural detail, is a challenge.

LB = DECORATOR/PATIENT

5th April 2022

WhatsApp group from decorator/patient

Photos. Just downed a Whitstable rock oyster in the Lobster Shack – hope it stays down! Now for the lobster thermidor.

5th April 2022

WhatsApp group – don't drink and decorate

Some responses:

Will

Looks great Grandad although some sunshine wouldn't be the worst thing…

Paul

Who else zoomed in to see if that was Dad in the sea? [This is re. a photo taken outside the Tate of Gormley's life-size standing statue appearing in the sea as the tide goes out!]

Anna

Stepping out – the world is slowly expanding…

5th May 2022

WhatsApp group from decorator/patient

We have just met the trauma team consultants. Those odds have improved again and are now 95:5. They want to see if I sink or swim in Greece before they discharge me and want to see holiday photos… They suggested I wear the dreaded boot for the journey and they seemed to want to come with us. This is not surprising when you see the clinic waiting room – I am now beginning to think I got off lightly. So, we are off to Greece on the 24th May – yippee!

5th May 2022

WhatsApp group – don't drink and decorate

Some responses:

Jane

Amazing news Dad – the Greek sun and food will do you so much good.

Lauren

Oh Grandad – that's amazing news.

Sarah

Wonderful news – watch out Greece…

Paul

Brilliant news Dad – a massive well done to you, Rosie and the team of experts.

Joe

That's great Grandad.

Kieran

Wonderful – whoohooo! He's back in action.

Beryl

Fantastic – so pleased you can go to Greece.

Jo

The very best news – so happy for you.

Anna

Such great news.

LB = DECORATOR/PATIENT

23rd May 2022

Email to Dear Susan from decorator/patient

Dear Susan – hope this finds you well – one final favour, please? I would appreciate it if you could forward this email to Mr Consultant. It is a last word from one of his patients who has had time to tell!

(This Dear Consultant email is included in Chapter 9 and Dear Susan's reply below).

23rd May 2022

Email from Dear Susan to decorator/patient

Dear Leonard

Mr Consultant thanks you for your thoughts and feedback. He wishes you well for your swim. Susan

24th May 2022

Email to Dear Susan from decorator/patient

Dear Susan

Thank you for your email of 23/5/22

Gatwick was mayhem until my surgical boot was spotted. I was then swept along with the disabled, had a yellow ribbon/label put round my neck and taken by special transport to an amazing lift contraption to be loaded/ boarded before luggage, babies, and the ambulant after which my walking stick was taken off me. Until ditto at Kalamata!

I attach a photo of the harbour wall!

24th May 2022

WhatsApp group from decorator/patient

The Eagles have landed and it's beautiful and hot.

We wish you were all here but we will manage!

25th May 2022

Email from Dear Susan to decorator/patient

So glad everything went well amongst the 'mayhem'. The harbour view looks very peaceful. Have a lovely time and hope you have amazing weather.

Susan

14th June 2022

Email to Dear Susan from decorator/patient

Dear Susan

Three weeks into my four-week trip to Greece (sorry!) I have today completed my swim to the harbour wall from the town beach...

Kind regards

14th June 2022

Email from Dear Susan to decorator/patient

Oh well done. It sounds like you are having a lovely time. Hope the weather is good. Enjoy the last week.

Susan

Chapter 11

Dear Secretary of State

Department of Health and Social Care London

14th September 2022

Dear Secretary of State

An outline blueprint for the NHS (which has been staring us in the face!)

We are not even sure you will ever get to see/read this but...!

We believe someone in your office should see/read this letter and study its attachments, which we have peddled around since soon after the Covid outbreak in 2020. These attachments form an outline blueprint that follows on from decades of work undertaken by your predecessors and numerous people at the department at great expense to the taxpayer. It is only now that its relevance to the current difficulties facing the NHS has become clear. It is too difficult a concept to be carried forward by the NHS and can only be actioned by your department. Hopefully someone will see how this kind of blueprint could compliment the rollout of the 160 community diagnostic centres being set up to diagnose patients quickly. This recent initiative needs the back-up of a progressive hospital service.

You will need to shortcut the cumbersome process currently in place to procure hospital buildings on an ad hoc basis which looks to reinvent the wheel for every project. It is time for your department to take control of this process and face up to the obvious need to provide the NHS with new healthcare facilities quickly starting with trauma and elective care specialities. The NHS's inadequate stock of existing hospital buildings is a major obstacle to a much-needed change of strategy.

This outline blueprint was included in our 'Evidence to the Health and Social Care Committee', dated 3rd September 2021. This suggested that the design of new hospitals has a direct bearing on how the NHS might recover from its own trauma, cope with the vaccine-shackled virus from now on, and get to grips with the massive backlog caused by the pandemic. Perhaps not unreasonably, the committee's interest was restrained – it was an exceptionally busy time and the issue of resource allocation in healthcare is perhaps too complex.

Also, you will see from our attachments that we tried to engage with the Epsom and St Helier University Hospitals NHS Trust re. a new hospital at Sutton (our brochure) and St George's University Hospital re. a new trauma centre. These approaches, as expected, were unsuccessful – clearly it is easier to ignore the substantial changes now needed to improve the NHS after the pandemic and to limp on doing what went before. This is the crux of the matter!

We do not need to be hear back from you. This outline blueprint and its intellectual property belongs to your department. We are now almost too old and exhausted to care and have done our bit! We just wish that someone could just get on with using this or something like it for the sake of the NHS and the people waiting to be treated and provided with a responsive service.

Now is the time to stop planning those too few, redundant large/mega hospitals and to get on with fixing the NHS by building many smaller, smarter, hospitals quickly in the right place...

Yours sincerely

LB and RG

Dear Secretary of State did not get in touch – ships had passed in the night! This secretary of state was reshuffled to another berth in Mr Sunak's first cabinet which seems hardly surprising. Also, no one in their right mind would expect that the replacement secretary of state would delve into the pending tray of a short-lived predecessor! This provoked the thought to write this book.

Perhaps no secretary of state or their numerous support staff would think that there could be a decorator/patient/retired architect and Rosemary out there who might be able to suggest using what had gone before to lever out a blueprint from the wealth of published guidance. A blueprint that might work today following the Covid-19 pandemic.

In a nutshell, NHS staff have the skills needed and there are probably enough of them trained up and ready to start all over again even though many feel they have had enough. However, most of the time they have the wrong vehicle to change speed, break new ground and to help drive forward a new strategy.

Surely this should be of interest to someone in 2023 – a year of NHS staff discontent?

Chapter 12
Enough is Enough

'Head in the clouds and feet on the ground.'

The most recent exchanges with Dear Susan and the WhatsApp group, 'don't drink and decorate' provide a fitting final chapter following the long road to recovery:

> 19th August 2022
>
> WhatsApp group – from decorator/patient:
>
> Sorry for the delay in reporting back following yesterday's appointment at St George's but sometimes silence is golden...
>
> However, prompted by a general need to know, it seems that it is still going to plan – it is just a long time coming. The orthopaedic man's work is done and dusted and his plastics sidekick wants to see us in two months if/when in the UK.
>
> Also, they both think we should keep up the good work, take as many holidays as we can, swim to the harbour wall as many times as possible, go on long walks, lose weight, drink less, cancel our birthdays from now on, keep jolly and cram in as many family visits as we can when we are not away on holiday.
>
> So, there you have it – life begins again like Michael Finnegan – begin again?

LB = DECORATOR/PATIENT

18th October 2022

WhatsApp group – from decorator/patient:

I am speaking very quietly – it's 2:30am, dark, damp and cold and we are waiting for Bob. He will ferry us to Gatwick so we can fly to Kalamata arriving 11am Greek time and there on to feel warm sunshine on our backs – so cheerio for now, all lovelies.

We leave you with a quote from Luciano Spalleti – newly appointed coach of Napoli.

'I had some time at home and there it is easy; you are with family. You walk a lot and strengthen your feet. And since there is a long way to go, having strong feet is a beautiful thing.'

So, thank you Luciano – whatever you all do please take care of your feet. Bob is here – yippee we're off!

20th October 2022

Email to Dear Susan from decorator/patient:

Dear Susan

Just in case Mr Consultant and Mr Consultant are wondering what on earth has become of me during the long gap between visits to the Orthoplastic clinic, I am in Greece again and it's wonderful.

I hope this finds you well.

Cheers.

28th October 2022

Email from Dear Susan to decorator/patient:

Hope you are having a relaxing break. Bring some sunshine back.

Susan

4th November 2022

Email to Dear Susan from decorator/patient:

Dear Susan

I am now back in the UK after a lovely relaxing break in Greece where the weather was perfect every day.

Already, I am settling into the familiar routine of cancelled outpatient appointments. My 17th November appointment was cancelled until 15th December, which was then cancelled until 19th January 2023. This has now been rearranged for April 2023.

What I am wondering of course is how this relates to my treatment regime and by what means consultants can possibly know how I am progressing without seeing me. So, I am emailing you to provide my own self-diagnosis for the hospital records.

It is tempting to say, after two years as an orthopaedic patient, that I am fixed. I have got off my bed and walked – maybe with an exaggerated limp but thanks to the orthopaedic team I still have my right leg...

The ulcer has cleared from my ankle and swelling is kind of under control. If I do a daily compression wrap, elevate when swelling occurs for at least a couple of hours a day, and stop wanting to climb every mountain and ford every steam I can still enjoy Greece and occasionally swim to the harbour wall...

There you have it – I am up and walking with no further need to attend St George's ever again. Please thank Mr Consultant and his team for all their efforts during what must have been the worst period for the NHS and St George's. A bouquet of flowers to them all and a special thank you for putting up with my frequent emails.

LB = DECORATOR/PATIENT

4th November 2022

Email from Dear Susan to decorator/patient:

Good morning

Hope you are well and thank you for the update which I have forwarded to Mr Consultant. Glad you are back safely and quite an achievement with all the walking at both airports. Keep well.

Susan

As expected, Mr Consultant was silent. 'Enough is enough' and greater needs must now be met.

It has been nearly three years since an alarming time was had by everybody as Covid pressurised the NHS. Also, it is more than two years down the road for the decorator/patient which has left him up and walking, albeit in the slow lane. His journey is here for all to read but it is necessary to stress how thankful he is to all those mentioned in despatches – and more.

However, no matter how thankful one is, it is easy to believe that nowadays admission to the NHS for treatment is nothing but a lottery. Some win and some lose. Clearly there can be no guarantees given for treating injuries or ill health but much more could be done to encourage organisational competence in buildings that are fit for purpose.

If hospital buildings transmit a feeling of obsolescence and neglect by the way they are planned and by looking badly maintained it will affect staff motivations, morale, patients' confidence, and often get in the way of treatment and a timely recovery. In some hospitals it is difficult not to want to be discharged soon after you are admitted because a downward spiral of unwellness and helplessness overcomes you in addition to what is expected after a surgical or medical procedure. A concern for patients' privacy, better meals, cleaner wards, with nurses and other staff more able to be alert to a patients' needs would all improve the patients' experience. These improvements must go hand in hand with a therapeutic approach to care and treatment in efficiently run facilities where patients can feel confident about what ls happening to them and why.

The aim should be to reduce admissions to as short a period as possible. This can be helped by providing hospitals that meet improved standards not far short of what one would expect from a good hotel. Better hospitals with the latest no-expense-spared equipment could help increase the turnover of patients using staff already in the NHS and help improve outcomes. Hospitals should be built to help save lives.

Everything about the NHS is too big to handle. It is time to downsize and for all users to feel able to feel part of something that is tangible. To help achieve this, there surely can be nothing better than to build new, easy, smart, smaller, 2020s hospitals quickly so that 'enough' becomes 'much more' and confidence in the NHS can be fully restored.

As of Friday 9th December 2022, seven million people were waiting on the NHS for a surgical or medical procedure.

END

PS BBC News – 11 December 2022

Edited by Jeremy Gahagan

Prof. Stephen Powis – NHS England also says we are now entering a fifth wave of Covid – adding it will take several years to get on top of the backlog created by the pandemic.

And Labour's Wes Streeting doesn't expect the doctors' union, the BMA, to treat him like 'some sort of heretic' for expecting services to improve for patients.

Also, from Wes Streeting, 'I want to get this right for patients. The NHS is so broken, we do have to think radically' – *The Times*, 7th January 2023.

'Public satisfaction with the NHS has slumped to its lowest level ever recorded. Just 29% said they were satisfied with the NHS in 2022 with waiting times and staff shortages the biggest concerns' – British Social Attitudes Survey, 29th March 2023.

Addendum

Fantasy Smaller Hospitals

After the worst of Covid, the NHS now must deal with a constant flow of emergencies and a massive backlog of less urgent but significant injuries and illnesses that are crippling the population. A new strategy is required. This could provide a rapidly built new generation of major trauma centres and elective care centres. Also, it could provide a range of other rapidly built centres like accident centres, women and children centres, chronic care centres, centres for elderly care, rehabilitation centres, cancer care centres, renal centres, and so on, in new, fast, easy, smart, smaller, hospitals. However, the immediate need is for trauma and elective care surgical centres. These can be built to sidestep what went before and what is going on now to inappropriately transform larger, failing, older hospitals, many of which are of the wrong time and are now in the wrong place. All specialties other than trauma and elective day care could continue to use suitable and better maintained existing hospitals like the last generation of nucleus hospitals until they also need replacing with new smaller hospitals.

What would a network of new, easy, fast, smart, smaller, hospitals all have in common given that, for example, major trauma centres and elective care centres are in many ways quite a different beast? Also, some way down the line it might also be necessary to build new smaller hospitals for other specialties.

Fantasy smaller hospitals should be:

- Able to be built quickly.
- Built and equipped to stand-alone, located where they are needed
- Uncomplicated, understandable, and flexible.
- No larger than 10,000 square metres.
- No higher than 4 stories high.
- Should have standardized/interchangeable suites, e.g., theatre suite, X-ray suite, etc.
- Smaller than 100 bedrooms (max) for an inpatient hospital – provided with mostly single and some double bedrooms all with ensuites, except in ITU.
- More like a hotel than a hospital.
- Accessible to air and road ambulances.
- Not able to be extended.
- Replaced when they become obsolete and as soon as someone thinks of extending them badly.
- Therapeutic and inspire confidence.
- Able to provide free and accessible parking.
- Accessible by rail and good public transport.

The above criteria could fit both trauma care and elective care, and all other specialties.

The major trauma centre would be 'open all hours' and could be fully planned and equipped with suites for emergency triage, X-ray, two or four theatre suites plus recovery and intensive care, rehabilitation, consultation/

orthoplastic clinic, i.e., be totally self-sufficient for treating trauma and for the long road to recovery. It would have mostly single bedrooms with ensuites except in recovery or intensive care spaces. It would have 64 bedrooms (max) in two wards. The 32-bedroom wards could be divided into four by eight-bedroom clusters (patients might choose to leave their wide doors open if they really want to be jolly or supportive!). These eight-room clusters might be allocated for high and medium dependency or women only, men only, children, older people, specialist treatment groups, or allocated randomly. It could be that a mix of single and double bedrooms might be provided to allow a spouse/partner/carer to stay with an adult patient who is needing their assistance or a parent to stay with an unwell child. Surely not too much to ask of an efficient future health service aiming to reduce how long a patient needs to stay.

Major trauma centres might be located not necessarily on existing hospital sites but where they are needed, say around the M25 or along other motorways connected by air ambulance and fast road ambulance services with a mainline railway station within spitting distance.

The elective care centre, being a day-care facility, would be 'open from 7am 'til midnight'. It too would be fully planned and equipped with suites for reception, X-ray, more theatres and recovery suites than an inpatient hospital as beds will not be needed, comfortable lounges for second stage recovery, rehabilitation, consultation/clinics. This too would be totally self-sufficient for day-care procedures.

Elective care centres could be located alongside trauma centres or be sited to be more accessible for local communities if necessary on an existing hospital site but self-contained and to stand alone to be managed separately from the existing hospital. Elective care centres should be accessible to air ambulances as well as road ambulances and public transport.

A network of fantasy smaller hospitals should have linked communications to manage movement of staff, supplies, and patient admissions.

As mentioned in the introduction, the decorator/patient/retired architect hoped that by the time he retired every hospital would be fit for purpose. He thought that at some time in the not-too-distant future the NHS would need fewer beds in smaller hospitals. These would be bright, shiny, optimistic, and therapeutic machines for healing which are full of hope and promise. Less staff would be doing so much more to mend/cure any condition/symptom and reduce the need for lengthy hospital admissions. A quick turnround of patients and a community support network with direct communication to these smaller hospitals would put right without fuss any mishap on the journey to a long and fit life.

Fantasy or wishful thinking maybe, but the Covid-19 pandemic has left an opportunity to change things using much of what is already available and already in place in the NHS. A touch on the rudder is needed to quickly straighten things out and to stop the NHS from going round and round in circles.

Nucleus hospitals now are a thing of the past. At that time some people thought they were too prescriptive, and many found its level of standardisation difficult, preferring a bespoke solution for each service. They argued that standardisation stifled creativity on individual schemes. Sadly, some of these individual schemes had square wheels. Nucleus met many of its challenges but on looking back it maybe was too big a hammer to crack a nut.

In 1975, when promoting nucleus hospitals, the health minister said, 'The NHS had in many areas not achieved the benefits from being a centralised service.' Maybe in the 2020s it might be appropriate to argue again for an element of standardisation so that the two key areas of need might be met by providing new, fast, smarter, smaller, hospitals using the latest technology for trauma care and elective care based on the criteria set out above. This might get the bull/NHS by the horns, leaving all other services to creatively determine how they use all existing hospitals needing an upgrade until they too feel a need to get on a smaller hospital bandwagon. We are talking here about a new start in providing efficient facilities for surgery to alleviate the pain and discomfort of so many people – and quickly.

Enough could be much more – someone should get on with it! Are there no longer lively clever Under-Secretaries in the Department of Health and Social Care or somewhere else in the Civil Service like the Treasury to tell their political masters and their advisors to stop sitting on their hands? They should be looking for medium-term strategies that can start to be delivered

LB = DECORATOR/PATIENT

quickly to get the NHS out of its deep hole and deal with the nation's health issues.

Once upon a time, on 30th April 1984, a letter was sent out from the Department of Health and Social Security. Extracts are included here to show that it was/is possible to take necessary action to point a finger at those people needing a kick up their backsides if there is a political will to make a real change.

> To
>
> Regional Administrators District Administrators
>
> Secretaries of the Special Health Authorities Secretaries of Boards of Governors
>
> For Action.
>
> Dear Administrator
>
> HOSPITAL BUILDING - NUCLEUS DESIGN SYSTEM
>
> 1. Ministers are concerned that, in some cases, health authorities are giving insufficient consideration to the advantages of using the Nucleus system for hospital design. Therefore, this letter reinforces capital planning procedures to ensure that health authorities take full account of the advantages of the Nucleus system when formulating proposals for building schemes.
>
> 2. The Nucleus system has been used successfully in England and Wales; nine Nucleus schemes are open; eleven schemes are at the construction or commissioning stage and several are at the design stage. Many other schemes have been influenced by the Nucleus approach.
>
> 3. ...

4. Health authorities are asked, in all cases, to consider Nucleus as a design option.

5. Where use of Nucleus is rejected a clear justification, based on service and site considerations, must be included in Approval in Principle or Budget Cost Submissions.

6. ...

7. ...

Yours sincerely

Under Secretary

Nationwide action can sometimes deliver!

Nucleus was stopped in its prime for reasons covered in earlier chapters but mainly because in-house expertise was put out to grass in an out-house agency that never could see the wood for the trees. Does this sound all too familiar?

Omission

The decorator/patient/retired architect decided not to include any designs and sketches in this book apart from the one inserted in Chapter 3 – to lighten the story and for old times' sake. This is even though there is mention of a brochure in correspondence included in emails to Dear Chairman, Dear Chief Transformation Officer, and Dear Mr Consultant. He has found over many years that the people best placed to change policy and implement new strategies tend to turn a blind eye at the sight of a plan or drawing. This can be no matter how diagrammatic or coloured up the presentation might be and how enthusiastic the presenter. It is therefore hardly surprising that the NHS is struggling with a failing estate. This book attempts to play a word game to avoid a need for illustrations.

Many healthcare professionals would find drawings depicting a smaller 100-bed hospital as complicated and hard to comprehend as a larger 800-bed version. You can see just how difficult it is for some people to understand plans by visiting any hospital. A variety of hit-and-miss brightly coloured way finder maps and signposting can be seen to cause chaos and confusion especially in large hospitals.[8]

---

[8] If this is thought to be an exaggeration try locating Hardy Ward at Kingston Hospital without finding yourself in the operating suite and ITU.

LB = DECORATOR/PATIENT

The intention with this book is to keep it simple and to try to describe some of the difficulties facing the NHS and a possible remedy. WhatsApp messages, emails, and letters are used to paint a picture about time spent in a very large St George's Hospital and an imaginary concept of a smaller hospital. It is the turn of others to illustrate how smaller hospitals should be designed and how they might look.

The Addendum takes a stab at setting out what might be considered as the criterion for a smaller hospital without using illustrations.[9] A process to realise smaller hospitals is set out in Chapter 8 in the evidence to the Health and Social Care Committee. This calls for a formal bidding structure/competition to be put in place with the expectation that it should involve the setting up of a specialist control group of healthcare professionals with a special interest in planning and hospital building design – as there was for Nucleus once upon a time.

---

[9] A louder voice is needed to argue the case for a buildings-led initiative for the NHS. It is highly unlikely that this will come from most architects who usually have to wait to be asked and then are expected to do as they are briefed. There are some architectural practices out there who are bursting to design a high-tech responsive future hospital and some when leading their field internationally have never had an opportunity to design a relevant ground breaking healthcare building for the NHS (Like Rogers, Foster, Hadid, and Grimshaw – what a difference these and some of the bright younger practices might make given half a chance!). Given the kind of challenge set out in this book, they could help lead a control group of healthcare professionals to design new facilities that look beyond the traditional mindset for the procurement of hospital buildings and help the NHS to take a massive leap forward to do what it does best in looking after the health of the nation.

A short letter to the RIBA journal

Horrible hospitals

Re 'Medical mutations' (RIBAJ, July, p38): I am not sure whether Christopher Shaw is speaking on behalf of Architects for Health or offering a personal view but my own opinion is that, following the first bout of Covid-19, we should avoid building 'European super hospitals' just as we should avoid if possible Covid-19. We should use those many hospital sites he mentions to build smarter, smaller hospitals that people (patients, their visitors and staff) can confidently access when they have to. These should be as unlike the nightmarish Nightingale hospitals as possible.

A large hospital is too big for patients and staff to comprehend and cannot be patient-focussed because its maze of rooms and corridors misinform, disorientate, and increase dependency. When it facilitates bad practice, it is not easily changed and because of its size and complexity, almost impossible to replace. Large hospitals have always become obsolete too soon and unmanageable for too long. We have had decades to understand this in project after project.

Len Bartholomew (former hospital planner and former member of Architects for Health)

August 2020

Acknowledgements and Epitaph

To all multidisciplinary teams who worked on the Nucleus Hospital Building Programme which was the purple patch of NHS Design Guidance for three decades. This data is still used as a benchmark. It was always intended to be used to promote change and innovation. All the many people involved thought that national guidelines were crucial for a better and fairer NHS.

Also, thanks to the late:

Howard Goodman

Percy Ward

Brian Hitchcox

Under Secretary 1984

Sheila Scott

Phillip Powell

Peter Skinner

Richard Burton

Danuta Blasczczyk

Jane Lamb

Tony Jones

Ron Graham

Natalie Slier

Maurice Fillery[10]

And the not so late:

Minister of State for Health 1975

Mike Meager

Geoff Mayers

Mike Singh

Don Eastwood

John Hall

John Meek

---

[10] Maurice James Fillery was moved from the 'And not so late' column to the 'Also, thanks to the late' column during the publication of this book. He died in the A&E at Kingston Hospital on 11th February 2023.

Maurice had been out of hospital for just over a week after four weeks as an inpatient in the same hospital. He firmly believed that he had outstayed his welcome as an inpatient and predicted he would have 'an untimely departure from this world within two weeks.' Maurice felt that he had been allowed to deteriorate by the hit-and-miss business of inpatient care of older people (or lack of it) and the appalling GP service over the last two years and just before admission. He was right on all counts.

Maurice was an intelligent man with many interests and complexities who should have been listened to – even though he was 94! Thankfully there are still some people alive to appreciate his contribution. We can now only listen to the sound of his silent protest.

Bill Simpson

Jonathan Millman

Stuart Robinson

Simon Mills

Judy Nolan (McTaggart)

Colin Gillert

Mungo Smith

Justin De Syllas

Ian Simpson

David Hutchison

Chris Pawley

Ian Wells

Robert Scott

The St George's major trauma team

St George's X-Ray department

The St George's chief transformation officer

District and GP practice nurses

The chairman of the Parliamentary Health and Social Care Committee 2020-2022

And uncle Tom Cobbley and all!

And last but not least – Dear Susan

LB = DECORATOR/PATIENT

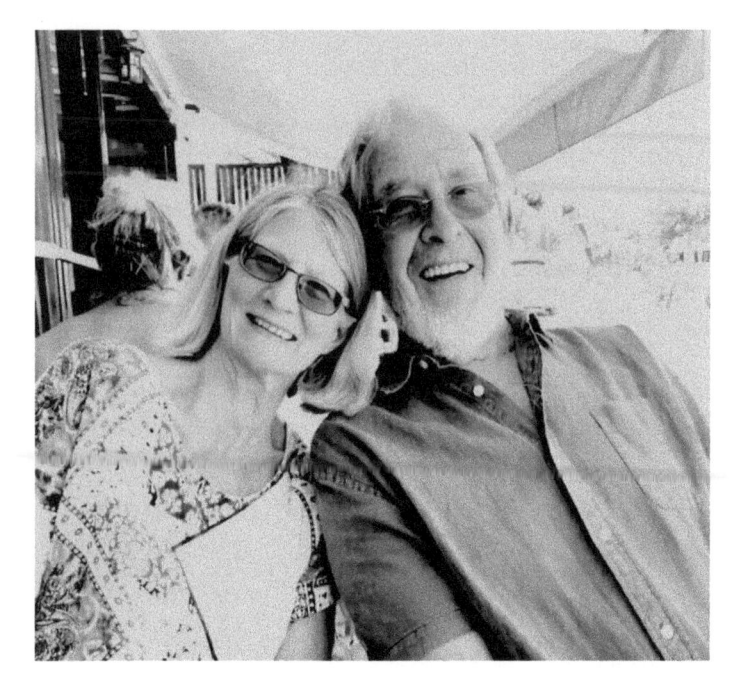

RG and LB out and about in Greece –
not too far from the harbour wall.

Over many years, they have had access to much of the Policy and Health Building documentation produced to guide the NHS.

Without the pandemic and a recent spell in hospital for LB, they too would not have bothered to think about what might be done to help the NHS.

A Last Word

BBC news – 17th May 2023 – Catherine Burns and Vicki Loader

Building work is yet to start for 33 of the Government's 40 promised new hospitals in England, the BBC has found.

Ministers aimed to have six ready for 2025 – but none of this group has full planning permission or funding yet.

Of the 40 hospitals on the list, eight were projects already planned.

One of the six due to be completed in 2025 is Epsom and St.Helier University Hospitals NHS Trust in Surrey.

A Department of Health and Social Care official said "We remain committed to delivering all 40 new hospitals by 2030 as part of the biggest hospital-building programme in a generation".

The new hospital programme is developing a new national approach to building these hospitals across England – and a standard approach should mean a more rapid process.

"We now need to plan our future hospital development on the basis of making essential provision for acute services in a way that will not pre-judge the eventual size of the district general hospitals. Fashions change: what is the conventional wisdom today may not be the wisdom of tomorrow. By building for the essential, not the desirable number of beds, one can spread the limited capital resources and start more new hospital development."

"The concept of the very large district general hospital has been increasingly, and in my view rightly, criticised. Large hospitals frequently have to be sited on the outskirts of towns and cities and are difficult to reach by public transport. There has been criticism about large hospitals because of their impersonal institutional nature for both staff and patients. Even economists have not been convinced by the arguments relating to economies of scale, some people claiming there are certain diseconomies of scale which operate in large hospitals."

Key note speech – Minister of Health, December 1975

I thought it worth finishing this book with the above quotes to help promote a new hospital building-led strategy. I am still convinced by these words and you should be too.

However, the passage of time has moved us further away from over-sized, unworkable, large district hospitals towards mega-hospitals. Small hospitals, built to target and face up to the backlog/waiting list following Covid, are needed now to revitalise the NHS.

LB
May 2023

Ingram Content Group UK Ltd.
Milton Keynes UK
UKHW010640200723
425492UK00004B/212